Women in Surgery

Kahyun Yoon-Flannery • Asanthi Ratnasekera
Maureen D. Moore

Editors

Women in Surgery

Navigating Challenges and Triumphs

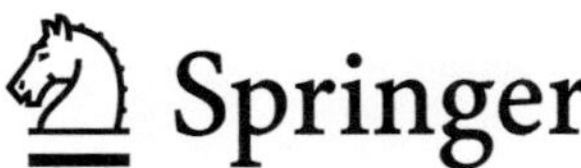 Springer

Editors
Kahyun Yoon-Flannery
Chief of Women's Cancer Services,
Chief of Breast Surgery
Atlanticare Regional Medical Center
Egg Harbor Township, NJ, USA

Asanthi Ratnasekera
Associate Trauma Medical Director,
Assistant Professor of Surgery
Christiana Care
Newark, DE, USA

Maureen D. Moore
Assistant Professor of Surgery,
Department of Surgery
Cooper University Hospital, Cooper
Medical School of Rowan University
Camden, NJ, USA

ISBN 978-3-032-10970-5   ISBN 978-3-032-10971-2   (eBook)
https://doi.org/10.1007/978-3-032-10971-2

This Springer imprint is published by the registered company Springer Nature Switzerland AG
The registered company address is: Gewerbestrasse 11, 6330 Cham, Switzerland

If disposing of this product, please recycle the paper.

Maureen D. Moore, MD

This book is dedicated to the two most important men in my life—My husband and my dad for all their sacrifice and love. I would like to also acknowledge my co-editors—thank you for the laughs and inspirations.

"Have the inner courage to each day say 'I will'." —John M. Daly, MD

Asanthi Ratnasekera, DO

This book is dedicated to all the powerful and strong women in my life. Women who pushed me to work hard and who taught me resilience, especially my late mother.

Kahyun Yoon-Flannery, DO

For my daughter, Aurelia Flannery, who is the most brilliant woman I have ever known and had the privilege to bring into this world. Life may not always be kind, but with her brilliance, resilience, and spark of defiance, she will always find her way. I am forever grateful to be her mother and partner in navigating all life's challenges.

Preface

As a woman surgeon long dedicated to advancing gender equality in medicine, I am beyond thrilled for the release of *Women in Surgery*. There is an old adage in surgery—that women can be harsh toward one another. While I have been fortunate to have both male and female mentors throughout my career, I have also faced moments shaped by misunderstanding and a lack of basic courtesy. Navigating multiple pregnancies during medical school, surgical residency, and early faculty years, I experienced firsthand the weight of preconceived notions and the challenges that come with defying them.

As a PGY-2 pregnant for the second time, I struggled to balance the demands of training with the realities of being a young mother. Many days passed without a sip of water, let alone a meal. To avoid delaying my eventual graduation, I used all my vacation days as "maternity leave," meaning I worked until the day I delivered. Scheduling calls became increasingly complicated. At the start of my third trimester—when exhaustion became my constant companion—I received a call from my scheduling chief: *"When exactly are you delivering this baby?"*

I was stunned. Not because I was defiant, but because the question itself revealed how little room our system allowed for humanity, from a woman to another woman. How could I possibly predict when my baby would arrive? Thankfully, another senior female resident stepped in and volunteered to cover my calls as backup should I go into labor unexpectedly. I ultimately went into labor early—after a 24-hour call at our busiest hospital—and my baby spent several days in the NICU. I finished my call and made it to my OB appointment 7 centimeters dilated.

Looking back, it's hard to believe this story could have been reality. My own residents today might think this is exaggerated. But that was the culture then: junior residents did not question orders; they simply endured. I often wish that the system had been built to better protect me, my baby, and my colleagues—to allow a small space of grace and anticipation around what should have been a joyous occasion.

This book is therefore dedicated to all who show up every day—the tireless surgical residents, the surgeons, the physicians—who give their all in the hospital while still maintaining their roles at home as mothers, wives, daughters, and partners. It is for every woman who wears many hats: doing it all exceptionally well on most days and simply surviving on others.

Egg Harbor Township, NJ, USA   Kahyun Yoon-Flannery, DO, FACS

Contents

Contributors

Tanya Anand, MD, MPH, FACS Clinical Assistant Professor of Surgery, Division of Trauma, Surgical Critical Care, Burns and Acute Care Surgery, Department of Surgery, University of Arizona, Tucson, AZ, USA

Vashti Bandy, MD Surgical Resident, Department of Surgery, Virginia Commonwealth University, Richmond, VA, USA

Amber Batool, DO, FACS, FACOS Assistant Professor of Surgery, Drexel University College of Medicine, Philadelphia, PA, USA

Vivian J. Bea, MD, MBA, FACS Section Chief of Breast Surgical Oncology, Department of Surgery, NewYork- Presbyterian Brooklyn Methodist Hospital, NewYork, NY, USA

Stephanie Bonne, MD, FACS, FCCM, FAMWA Professor of Surgery, Wake Forest University School of Medicine, Winston-Salem, NC, USA
Department of Surgery, Advocate Christ Medical Center, Oak Lawn, IL, USA

Karen Brasel, MD, MPH, FACS Vice President, American Board of Surgery, Philadelphia, PA, USA
Professor, Oregon Health & Science University, Portland, OR, USA

Lisa K. Cannada, MD, FAAOS, FAOA, FACS Adjunct Professor, Department of Orthopaedics, University of North Carolina, Chapel Hill, NC, USA
Director of Faculty Integration, UNC SOM Charlotte, Charlotte, NC, USA
Novant Health Orthopaedic Fracture Clinic, Charlotte, NC, USA

Margo Carlin, DO Department of Surgery, Christiana Care, Newark, DE, USA

Alexis Colley, MD, MS Department of Surgery, University of California San Francisco (UCSF), San Francisco, CA, USA

Madolyn Conant, BS Department of Surgery, University of Arizona, Tucson, AZ, USA

Marie Crandall, MD, MPH, FACS Richard B. Fratianne Professor of Surgery, Case Western Reserve University, Cleveland, OH, USA
Chair of Surgery, MetroHealth, Cleveland, OH, USA

Lucy M. De La Cruz, MD, FACS Chief of Breast Surgery, MedStar Georgetown University Hospital, Washington, DC, USA
Associate Professor of Surgery, Georgetown University School of Medicine, Washington, DC, USA

Beth B. Dupree, MD, FACS, ABOIM Redeemer Health, Southampton, PA, USA

Jacklyn M. Engelbart, MD, MSCI Department of Surgery, University of Iowa, Iowa City, IA, USA

Haley Eversman, BS Department of Surgery, University of Arizona, Tucson, AZ, USA

Betty Fan, DO, FACS Assistant Professor, Breast Surgery, Department of General Surgery, University of Chicago, Chicago, IL, USA

Genevieve A. Fasano, MD, MS Department of Surgery, Weill Cornell Medicine, New York, NY, USA

Paula Ferrada, MD, FACS, FCCM, MAMSE Chair, Department of Surgery Inova Fairfax Medical Campus, Falls Church, VA, USA
Medical Director Perioperative Services IFMC, Falls Church, VA, USA
Division and System Chief for Trauma and Acute Care Surgery Inova Healthcare System, Falls Church, VA, USA
Professor, University of Virginia School of Medicine, Charlottesville, VA, USA
ELAM class 2020, Falls Church, VA, USA

Carla Suzanne Fisher, MD, MBA, FACS Professor of Surgery, Chief, Division of Breast Surgery, Indiana University School of Medicine, Indianapolis, IN, USA

Nicole Fox, MD, MPH, FACS Professor of Surgery, Associate Chief Medical Officer, Cooper Medical School of Rowan University, Camden, NJ, USA
Cooper University Health Care, Camden, NJ, USA

Brianna R. Fram, MD Assistant Professor, Department of Orthopaedic Surgery and Rehabilitation Medicine, University of Chicago, Chicago, IL, USA

Amy J. Goldberg, MD, FACS Marjorie Joy Katz Dean, Lewis Katz School of Medicine at Temple University, Philadelphia, PA, USA

Katherine D. Gray, MD Assistant Attending Thoracic Surgeon, Memorial Sloan Kettering Cancer Center, New York, NY, USA

Alyssa Habermann, MD Surgical Resident, Department of Surgery, Virginia Commonwealth University, Richmond, VA, USA

Tatiana Hoyos Gomez, MD, FACS Assistant Professor, Oregon Health & Science University, Portland, OR, USA

Rebekah Huckeby, MD Division of Trauma, Surgical Critical Care, Burns and Acute Care Surgery, Department of Surgery, University of Arizona, Tucson, AZ, USA

Aditi M. Kapil, MD, FACS Assistant Professor of Surgery, Yale School of Medicine, New Haven, CT, USA

Elinore J. Kaufman, MD, MSHP, FACS Assistant Professor of Surgery, University of Pennsylvania, Philadelphia, PA, USA

Kristen Knapp, MD Department of Surgery, Cooper University Hospital, Cooper Medical School of Rowan University, Camden, NJ, USA

Lindsay E. Kuo, MD, MBA, FACS Associate Professor of Surgery, Lewis Katz School of Medicine, Philadelphia, PA, USA

Erika B. Lindholm, MD Assistant Professor of Pediatrics and Surgery, Division of Pediatric Surgery, Cooper University Hospital, Cooper Medical School of Rowan University, Camden, NJ, USA

Julie A. Margenthaler, MD, FACS Professor of Surgery, Division of General Surgery, Section of Surgical Oncology, Washington University in St. Louis, St. Louis, MO, USA

Kandace P. McGuire, MD, FACS Chief of Breast Surgery, Professor of Surgery, Department of Surgery, Virginia Commonwealth University, Richmond, VA, USA

Andrea M. Mesiti, MD Department of Surgery, Weill Cornell Medicine, New York Presbyterian Hospital, New York, NY, USA

Maureen D. Moore, MD, FACS Assistant Professor of Surgery, Department of Surgery, Cooper University Hospital, Cooper Medical School of Rowan University, Camden, NJ, USA

Neelam Mulji, MD Breast Surgical Oncology Fellow, MedStar Georgetown University Hospital, Washington, DC, USA

Marc A. Neff, MD Medical Director, Center for Surgical Weight Loss, Jefferson Health New Jersey, Cherry Hill, NJ, USA

Andrea Pakula, MD, MPH, FACS Medical Director of Robotic Surgery, Chair, Department of Surgery, General, Bariatric and Hernia Surgery, Trauma, Critical Care and Acute Care Surgery, Adventist Health, Roseville, CA, USA

Ashwini Paranjpe, MD Assistant Professor, Breast Surgical Oncology, Department of Surgery, Virginia Commonwealth University, Richmond, VA, USA

Pauline K. Park, MD, FACS, FCCM Professor of Surgery, Co-Director Surgical Intensive Care Unit, Program Director, Surgical Critical Care Fellowship, Department of Surgery, Division of Acute Care Surgery, University of Michigan, Ann Arbor, MI, USA

Mary Lou Patton, MD, FACS, FICS, FSSO, FCCM Emerita Professor of Surgery, MainLine Health, Formerly Crozer Health, Delaware, PA, USA

Mara A. Piltin, DO, FACS Vice Chair of Innovation, Department of Surgery, Assistant Professor of Surgery, Division of Surgical Oncology, Mayo Clinic, Rochester, NY, USA

Arunima Punjala, MD Surgical Resident, Department of Surgery, Virginia Commonwealth University, Richmond, VA, USA

Asanthi Ratnasekera, DO, FACS Associate Trauma Medical Director, Assistant Professor of Surgery, Christiana Care, Newark, DE, USA

Lisa M. Reid, MD, FACS Head, Section of Endocrine Surgery, Cooper University Hospital, Camden, NJ, USA

Sylvia A. Reyes, MD, MBS, FACS Director of Breast Services Health Equity Programs at Northwell Zuckerberg Cancer Center, Assistant Professor of Surgery, Zucker School of Medicine at Hofstra, Long Island, NY, USA

Mckenzie Rowe, MD Surgical Resident, Department of Surgery, Inova Fairfax Health, Falls Church, VA, USA

Rachel M. Russo, MD, MAS, NHDP-BC, FACS Veteran, USAF MC, Assistant Professor In Residence, Department of General Surgery, Division of Acute Care Surgery, UC Davis Health, Sacramento, CA, USA

Hannah M. Sadek, RN, AGACNP-BC Nurse Practitioner, Division of Acute Care Surgical Services, Virginia Commonwealth University Health, Richmond, VA, USA

Michelle C. Salazar, MD, MHS Thoracic Surgery Fellow, Memorial Sloan Kettering Cancer Center, New York, NY, USA

Tandis Soltani, MD Assistant Professor of Surgery, Division of Acute Care Surgery and Surgical Critical Care, Department of Surgery, Loma Linda University Health, Loma Linda, CA, USA

Julie Ann Sosa, MD, MA, FACS, FSSO Leon Goldman, MD Distinguished Professor of Surgery and Chair, Department of Surgery, Professor, Department of Medicine, Affiliated Faculty, Philip R. Lee Institute for Health Policy Studies, University of California San Francisco (UCSF), San Francisco, CA, USA

Jennifer F. Tseng, MD, MPH, FACS Professor of Surgery Emerita, Boston University, Boston, MA, USA
Clinical Professor of Surgery, Creighton University, Omaha, NE, USA

Amy Vertrees, MD Founder, Boss Business of Surgery Series, Columbia, TN, USA

Corinne Wee, MD Clinical Assistant Professor of Surgery, Division of Plastic and Reconstructive Surgery, Department of Surgery, MetroHealth Medical Center, Cleveland, OH, USA

Audrey R. Yang, BS Department of Surgery, University of Arizona, Tucson, AZ, USA

Heather L. Yeo, MD, MHS, MS, MBA Associate Professor of Surgery, Weill Medical College of Cornell University, New York, NY, USA

Kahyun Yoon-Flannery, DO, MPH, FACS Chief of Women's Cancer Services, Chief of Breast Surgery, AtlantiCare Regional Medical Center, Egg Harbor Township, NJ, USA

Part I
Historical Perspectives on Women in Surgery

Chapter 1
The Early Challenges: The Historical Perspective on Women in Surgery

Mary Lou Patton

As the sixth and last born at our home on the farm in 1947, I didn't realize initially how fortunate I was that my grandfather, in 1921, had an indoor bathroom added to the house. As for our family, my sister told me that after my twin brothers were born in 1944, the boys were considered very "special." Being three years younger, I never appreciated the differences in special treatment. I just always knew boys got more liberties in our family and community.

We raised animals and crops. All worked hard on the farm. In the 8th grade, our county school had closed the prior year, and forced to join the city school. I had gone from a class of 10–14 pupils with one teacher and having two to three grades in one room, to a class of 200 pupils with one teacher. In each class, topics were taught with 10–30 pupils. I had not given much thought before this about further education. Although my aunt had graduated from the Miami University of Ohio in the 1930s, Dad felt she never utilized her education to her advantage. He was not going to provide me with financial support. I began looking for the least expensive postsecondary education. I had wanted to be a math major at Ohio State University (OSU), where my dad and my brothers had gone. However, at the time, nursing school was the least expensive. Dad trashed my first response from a nursing school, "didn't want his daughter emptying bed pans" I contacted Miss Carroll, the director of Springfield City Hospital, Ohio, as a heads-up. She not only accepted my application but also provided me with a loan to be paid back after graduation.

During my rotation at Children's Hospital in Cincinnati, Ohio, I began considering medicine and continued the nursing program, more eager to learn than ever. After my graduation with honors, Miss Carroll strongly encouraged me to go to New York City for work. I started my first employment at the Columbia-Presbyterian

M. L. Patton (✉)
Emerita Professor of Surgery, Main Line Health, Formerly Crozer Health,
Delaware, PA, USA
e-mail: pattonmarylou@gmail.com

K. Yoon-Flannery et al. (eds.), *Women in Surgery*,
https://doi.org/10.1007/978-3-032-10971-2_1

Medical Center in NYC. I visited colleges and universities and decided on Columbia University. There was a 2-year requirement of a foreign language for graduation. I found speaking, writing, and taking dictation outrageously difficult, so I decided to go to Université de Paris to complete my requirement in language. It was a fun and exciting year.

I returned to New York City. At the end of the winter semester, I married, and in March, returned to Ohio with my husband. We completed our degrees, mine in pre-medicine, and I applied to medical schools. Ohio State, where my father and brother had gone, stated they "would not consider my application because I already had a career, nursing".

Fortunately, I got an interview from Harvard with Professor Malhek T. Rotman, MD. Although she was concerned that Harvard only accepted a few out-of-state applicants at this time, she suggested I move to Boston. Also, she gave me the names of other schools favorable to women. Arkansas program was known to accept women with children. At that time, my daughter, Nickie, was 2½ years old. Even better for our family at the time, my interviewer knew Dr. Mark Rayport at the Medical College of Ohio. I was interviewed and accepted. I had wanted to do their MD-PhD program, but one interviewer was adamant that I apply only for one or the other. I was accepted to the MD program.

During my surgical rotation in medical school, Dr. Robert T. Tidrick, who had previously, for 19 years, been the Chief of Surgery at Iowa University, exposed me to an exciting career in surgery. I was impressed by his bedside manner and the care he gave to the whole patient. In medical school, another student and I received the surgical award at graduation. Dr. Robert T. Tidrick felt the Iowa surgical program was a great fit for me since I was raised on a farm. In medical school, I was the only student who had been raised on a farm.

At the time in 1979, Iowa had matriculated only two women in its surgical residency program, one of whom was an emergency medicine attending and not a surgical attending. There was a research rotation for residents in their third year if they wanted. I did mine in the dog laboratory, and my work was published in a journal Circulatory Shock (volume 10, number 4, 10:317–327, 1985). I presented my work at the annual meeting of the Iowa Academy of Surgery in Ames, Iowa, on April 17th, 1982.

At one point, the Chief of Surgery in 1982–1983 decided I would not be allowed to complete the surgical residency program at Iowa. Dr. Tedrick gave me a position back in Ohio, where I went to medical school. However, it was decided that I could complete the Iowa surgical program.

In August 1984, I arrived in Wallingford, PA, and was to begin my career as an attending. I had arrived a month earlier than my start date to adjust and to spend time with my daughter and husband. The surgeon and soon-to-be Chief of Surgery, who hired me for burn care, was starting a project of cultured epithelial autografts (CEA). The project was completed by Dr. Howard Greer, the Chair of the Department of Physiology at Harvard, who spearheaded the final product. Our team used the CEA on a 50-year-old male with 90% burn wounds who survived. The process involved a biopsy of the patient and the cells grown in a laboratory, and then sent to our burn center for grafting in 1989. Dr. Basil Pruitt was skeptical and said he thought of the process as the fable "the emperor's clothing," but after seeing our patient, he rescinded his comment to me.

March 20, 1992, Dr. Linwood Haith and I were working on a project on extracorporeal membrane oxygenation (ECMO). Burn patients were dying of this disease, ARDS (adult respiratory distress syndrome). I visited Professor Luciano Gattinone in Milan, Italy, to learn his process and discuss our ARDS patients' results. Fellows and attendings managed the patients 24/7. Our team, especially Dr. Haith and I, had all the ins and outs completed with the plan and the paperwork for our patients. Our administration reviewed our detailed plan and how we would help cover expenses, but on re-review, they reported it was not financially possible. We then did the second best for us and developed an excellent relationship with an ECMO center in Philadelphia and published in *Burns* (24, 1998, 566–568) the first adult burn patient with ARDS treated with ECMO to survive. The patient returned to us, and we completed his burn wound care.

I was hired to provide burn care, but was expected and needed to, for financial purposes, develop my own general surgical career. I had an office originally at the end of a hallway of an empty, unused patient's room, which limited my access to referring physicians. My practice in general surgery (as it was) had not had time or place to develop. The surgery department was in the midst of developing a level 2 Trauma Center. The Chief of Surgery had me take most of the 24-h call for a year or two. I remember two distant cases: a gunshot wound to the chest and neck laceration, both requiring extensive repair, and finally a fall injury from a construction site with a significant splenic injury, but the patients were stable. I chose at that time to treat the patients with observation and received "a lot" of flak. Fortunately, the young man with the splenic injury did well, and this would now be an acceptable form of treatment.

In addition, there was pressure from the Chief to develop an endoscopy practice. I was locked out of the G.I. laboratory initially, so I purchased my own upper and lower G.I. endoscopes. I scoped at that time in my new office, which I rented, in the patient rooms in the hospital, and in our surgery unit and administered my own anesthesia.

I was informed by the Pentax representative that Dr. Gerard Marks, a nationally known colorectal surgeon and an expert in endoscopy, and I were the only surgeons who had purchased Pentax scopes in the Philadelphia area. In 1988, I presented Percutaneous Endoscopic Gastrostomy feeding tubes in burn patients at the Society of American Gastrointestinal and Endoscopic Surgeons (SAGES) in San Antonio, Texas. Later, it was published in *Surgical Endoscopy* (1994, September 8, 91:1067–71).

To boost the colonoscopy practice for general surgeons, I and eight other general surgeons published in the *American Journal of Surgery* (volume 163, 1992, pages 257–259) "Can general surgeons perform colonoscopy safely?". Our study of over 1000 cases showed that we compared favorably with postgraduate endoscopy fellowship-trained gastroenterologists. In 1994, I did a concomitant laparoscopic cholecystectomy and splenectomy for the surgical management of hereditary spherocytosis in a 16-year-old female and a few years later on her brother. My reported case was the first in the USA, *American Journal of Surgery* (1997 June; 66 (6): 536–539).

In another instance, a patient of mine insisted I repair his inguinal hernia laparoscopically. I told him I had never done one, so he told me, "then learn how because that's the only way I'm having it done". Fortunately, at that time, there was a conference in Bordeaux, France, and Dr. Lloyd Nyhus, a world-renowned hernia surgeon from the USA, who had favored the traditional open method was there. At our conference group, he said the success of laparoscopic hernia repair was hard to argue against. I went a workshop and learned how. The patient was pleased, and several years later, he called my office and wanted the other side done. In 1994, I was called to the OR by a gynecologist to see a pubic defect that we were able to identify as an obturator hernia. This was repaired, and it was reported to the *Journal of the Society of Laparoscopic Surgeons* (JSLS) (April 1988; 212:191–193). Only eight other cases had been reported in the international literature at that time.

As with most women surgeons in my time, we were pushed into practicing breast surgery specialty, even if that was not really appreciated by the male surgeons, at least at my institution. My grandmother had died of metastatic breast cancer the year before I was born, and I had heard so many distressing accounts in my young life that I was not at all anxious to do breast diseases. Interestingly, also in residency, the two male surgeons never allowed me to do a mastectomy, but I certainly retracted and 1st assisted in enough cases.

Early on in my career, half of my general surgical cases were breast. I became a Fellow of the International College of Surgeons (FICS) after presenting and publishing on breast disease in 1996 (breast conservative surgery with radiation treatment for women with stage TIS, 1, or 2 breast cancer). I presented at Washington, DC, during a conference on April 4th, 1996, and published in the *International College of Surgeons* (volume 81, number 4; October–December 1996). The cases spanned from 1987 to 1995.

In 1991, the National Institute of Health Consensus stated that breast conservation was an appropriate treatment for breast cancer versus mastectomy. However, breast conservation was not enthusiastically accepted until years later.

Thanks to the National Accreditation Program for Breast Centers (NAPBC), cases were reviewed, and surgeons who did not comply with biopsy first were rarely referred for breast cancer care from family doctors, oncologists, or medical doctors. It was before there were designations as breast centers by the NAPBC that our hospital had surgeons, radiologists, pathologists, oncologists, and radiation oncologists, meet weekly as a "breast panel" for conferences. We also had a tumor board weekly, too, but on a different time and day. I was the cancer liaison and a few years, co-director of the cancer committee. In 1995, I joined the American Society of Breast Surgeons. In 2002, I became a fellow in the Society of Surgical Oncology (FSSO), the first in Delaware County, Pennsylvania.

In 2008, the NAPBC commenced, and our program joined within the first few months of this initiation and continued throughout my career. In 2013, after being very active in breast care, I completed phases 1 and 2 at the City of Hope, Duarte, California, the "Intensive Course in Cancer Risk Assessment."

Never did I regret a day of my surgical career and the opportunity to teach hundreds of residents from the University of Pennsylvania, Jefferson, Drexel, Philadelphia College of Osteopathic Medicine, and Christiana Care, and how wonderful then to see the increase in women graduating from surgical residencies and women surgical attendings.

In 2022–2023, I was honored with the Who's Who of America (Marquis). The plaque states, to "individuals who possess professional integrity, demonstrates outstanding achievement in their respective fields and have made immense contribution to society as a whole."

Chapter 2
Pioneering Women in Surgery

Lindsay E. Kuo and Amy J. Goldberg

Women are a growing presence in general surgery and make up nearly one-quarter of the active general surgical workforce and nearly half of general surgery trainees [1, 2]. Today's female surgeons follow in the footsteps of numerous pioneers, who became surgeons when it was incredibly uncommon for women to become physicians, much less surgeons. Here, we explore the histories of a few of our notable pioneering female surgeons.

Mary Edwards Walker

Mary Edwards Walker is widely recognized as the first female surgeon. Born in 1832, she was the second female graduate of Syracuse Medical College in 1855 [3]. Following graduation, she attempted to establish a practice as a physician and surgeon, but was not successful as the public did not accept a female doctor. After the start of the Civil War in 1861, Dr. Walker volunteered to serve in the Union Army as a surgeon, but was denied a commission. Instead, she chose to serve as an unpaid civilian surgeon [4]. In 1863, she was appointed a surgeon by the Army, a position she served for the remainder of the war [3, 4]. For her service, she was awarded the Medal of Honor for Meritorious Service by President Andrew Johnson. Today, she remains the only female Medal of Honor recipient [5].

L. E. Kuo (✉)
Associate Professor of Surgery, Lewis Katz School of Medicine, Philadelphia, PA, USA
e-mail: Lindsay.kuo@tuhs.temple.edu

A. J. Goldberg
Marjorie Joy Katz Dean, Lewis Katz School of Medicine at Temple University, Philadelphia, PA, USA
e-mail: Amy.goldberg@tuhs.temple.edu

© The Author(s), under exclusive license to Springer Nature Switzerland AG 2026
K. Yoon-Flannery et al. (eds.), *Women in Surgery*,
https://doi.org/10.1007/978-3-032-10971-2_2

After the conclusion of the war, Dr. Walker advocated for women's rights. She was arrested numerous times for wearing pants and other clothes only worn by men at the time. In 1912 and 1914, Dr. Walker testified before the United States House of Representatives in support of women's right to vote [3, 4]. Her legacy is honored with the Mary Edwards Walker Inspiring Women in Surgery Award, which is presented yearly at the American College of Surgeons [6].

Margaret Chung

Born in 1889 to Chinese immigrant parents, Margaret Chung matriculated to the University of Southern California College of Physicians and Surgeons, graduating in 1916 [7]. She was the first Asian woman to graduate from medical school in the USA. Dr. Chung's goal was to become a medical missionary, but she was turned down due to her race. Instead, Dr. Chung entered into training in both surgery and medicine. After a few years, she took a position at the Santa Fe Railroad Hospital in Los Angeles. There, she began a surgical practice [8, 9]. In 1922, she relocated to San Francisco with the goal of introducing modern Western medicine to the immigrant Chinese population. In 1925, Dr. Chung became one of four inaugural department chairs at Chinese Hospital in San Francisco [7].

After the Japanese invasion of China in 1931, Dr. Chung volunteered to serve as a frontline surgeon but was turned down [7]. Instead, she was asked to recruit pilots from the United States to serve in China; subsequently, she also recruited soldiers and submariners. After the USA entered the war, Dr. Chung advocated for greater involvement of women in the military. Her efforts led to the establishment of the WAVES (Women Accepted for Volunteer Emergency Service), a reserve corps of female naval officers [7].

Dorothy Lavinia Brown

Born in Philadelphia in 1919, Dorothy Lavinia Brown attended Bennett College, a historically Black college or university (HBCU) in North Carolina, then Meharry Medical College, from which she graduated in 1948. After an intern year at Harlem Hospital, Dr. Brown completed a general surgery residency at Meharry in 1955. That same year, she became the first Black female surgeon fellow of the American College of Surgeons. Beginning in 1957, Dr. Brown was the Chief of Surgery at Riverside Hospital in Nashville, a position she held until 1983. It is thought that she was the first Black female surgeon, certainly in the South but perhaps nationally [10].

Dr. Brown's legacy extends beyond the world of surgery: she became the first single person to adopt a child in Tennessee. In 1966, Dr. Brown was elected to the Tennessee state legislature, the first Black woman to hold that position [10, 11]. She also helped pass the Negro History Act, mandating that Tennessee schools teach about the accomplishments of Black people [11]. In this role as a legislator, and throughout the remainder of her career, Dr. Brown fought for the rights of women and people of color.

Olga Jonasson

Olga Jonasson graduated from the University of Illinois College of Medicine in 1958, when just 6% of physicians were women. She then entered into a general surgery residency at the University of Illinois Research and Education Hospital and graduated in 1964. This was followed by fellowships in immunohistochemistry and transplant immunology, followed by a cardiovascular and thoracic surgery fellowship. Dr. Jonasson then became the first female transplant surgeon [12].

Dr. Jonasson continued to blaze a trail: in 1968, she established the division of transplantation at the University of Illinois at Chicago. Less than 10 years later, she became Chief of Surgery at Cook County Hospital, and in 1987, Dr. Jonasson became the Chair of Surgery at The Ohio State University [12]. In doing so, Dr. Jonasson became the first female Chair of an academic surgery department. Later in her career, Dr. Jonasson served as the inaugural Medical Director of the Education and Surgical Services division of the American College of Surgeons [13].

Beyond these notable accomplishments, Dr. Jonasson was renowned for her mentorship to countless students, residents, and faculty members [12, 13]. In her memory, the American College of Surgeons established in 2007 a yearly lecture in her honor [6].

Patricia Numann

Patricia Numann spent her entire surgical career at the State University of New York—Upstate, where she also trained, graduating from general surgery residency in 1970. Dr. Numann developed a practice focused on breast and endocrine surgery, establishing the first Comprehensive Breast Care Center in 1986. Dr. Numann also devoted much of her career to advancing surgical education: after founding the Association for Surgical Education, she also served as its President. Dr. Numann also served as President of the American College of Surgeons, the second woman to hold this seat, and was the first female Chair of the American Board of Surgery [14, 15].

Perhaps Dr. Numann's most lasting legacy, however, is her creation of the Association of Women Surgeons in 1981 [16]. That year, Dr. Numann invited female surgeons to breakfast at the annual meeting of the American College of Surgeons; the tradition continued yearly until the AWS was formally incorporated in 1986 [16]. Dr. Numann fittingly served as president that year. Since then, the Association of Women Surgeons (AWS) has grown nationally and internationally to support women surgeons at all phases of their careers.

Contemporary Pioneers: Jo Buyske and Patricia Turner

Two female surgeons currently stand out as national leaders in American surgery: Jo Buyske and Patricia Turner.

Jo Buyske is the CEO and President of the American Board of Surgery (ABS). Dr. Buyske first served as a Director of the ABS in 2006, followed by roles as Associate Executive Director and Director of Evaluation in 2008, and Executive Director in 2017. Prior to that service, Dr. Buyske was the Chief of Surgery and director of minimally invasive surgery at Penn Presbyterian Medical Center in Philadelphia. Dr. Buyske also sits as a director of the American Board of Medical Specialties [17].

Patricia Turner was named Executive Director of the American College of Surgeons in 2022, the first woman to serve in that position. Prior to that, she served as Director of the Division Member Services in the American College of Surgeons beginning in 2011. A trained minimally invasive surgeon, Dr. Turner is also an adjunct professor of surgery at the University of Chicago Pritzker School of Medicine. Dr. Turner was also the first female president of the Society of Black Academic Surgeons [18, 19].

In these roles—Dr. Buyske is overseeing certification of general surgeons through the ABS, and Dr. Turner is supporting surgeons and patients through the ACS—these two women are molding general surgery for the future. Both are exemplary role models for all surgeons, male and female alike.

Conclusion

Each of these women—and countless others—paved the way for today's female surgeons. Many also advanced the cause of women, or those who could not advocate for themselves, in other arenas. With these inspiring examples, we can all strive to achieve the same for generations to come.

References

1. "Women in Surgery: Increasing in Numbers – And Influence." Accessed June 3, 2025. https://rwjms.rutgers.edu/magazine/winter-2025/women-surgery-increasing-numbers-influence#:~:text=Nearly%20a%20quarter%20(22.6%20percent,and%20neurosurgery%20(10%20percent).
2. Kurapati SS, Moeckel C, Stegman MM, et al. A Flattened Curve: National Trends of Women Physicians and Residents in Surgery Over the Last Decade. J Surg Res 2024;303:506–512.
3. Accessed June 3, 2025. https://www.womenshistory.org/education-resources/biographies/mary-edwards-walker
4. Accessed June 3, 2025. https://www.nps.gov/people/mary-walker.htm

5. Accessed June 3, 2025. https://www.army.mil/article/183800/meet_dr_mary_walker_the_only_female_medal_of_honor_recipient
6. Accessed July 27, 2025. https://www.facs.org/about-acs/governance/acs-committees/women-in-surgery-committee/
7. Accessed June 2, 2025. https://www.nytimes.com/2023/09/18/obituaries/margaret-chung-overlooked.html
8. Accessed June 2, 2025. https://exhibits.stanford.edu/riseup/feature/dr-margaret-chung
9. Accessed June 2, 2025. https://www.nps.gov/people/dr-margaret-mom-chung.htm
10. Accessed June 1, 2025. https://cfmedicine.nlm.nih.gov/physicians/biography_46.html
11. Accessed June 1, 2025. https://www.facs.org/for-medical-professionals/news-publications/news-and-articles/bulletin/2022/04/trailblazing-women-minority-surgeons-dr-dorothy-l-brown-surgeon-legislator-and-teacher/
12. Sims CA, Leemaster J, Pawlik TM. Inspirational Women in Surgery: Olga Jonasson, the Legacy of the First Female to Chair an Academic Department of Surgery. World J Surg. 2021 Sep 2;46(4):755-756.
13. Accessed June 1, 2025. https://www.facs.org/about-acs/archives/past-highlights/jonassonhighlight/
14. Accessed June 2, 2025. https://www.amwa-doc.org/awards/blackwell-exhibit/patricia-joy-numann-md/
15. Accessed June 2, 2025. https://guides.upstate.edu/women-in-medicine/patricia-numann
16. Accessed June 2, 2025. https://www.womensurgeons.org/history
17. Accessed June 3, 2025. https://program.absurgery.org/default.jsp?aboutbios
18. Accessed June 3, 2025. https://www.facs.org/for-medical-professionals/news-publications/news-and-articles/bulletin/2021/07/patricia-l-turner-md-mba-facs-named-next-executive-director-of-the-acs/
19. Accessed June 3, 2025. https://en.wikipedia.org/wiki/Patricia_L._Turner

Chapter 3
Lessons from the Past: Paving the Way for Women in Surgery

Andrea M. Mesiti and Heather L. Yeo

Introduction

The demographics of surgery have changed dramatically over the years. Nearly half of current US surgical residents now identify as women, a welcome shift in a historically male-dominated field [9]. Looking back at the history of women in surgery reveals critical lessons that continue to shape the experiences of current and future surgeons. The resilience and passion demonstrated by early pioneers laid the foundation for ongoing efforts to diversify the field and address the unique challenges faced by women in surgery.

Resiliency

One of the most enduring lessons from early women surgical leaders is that of resilience. Historically, medicine—and surgery in particular—were unwelcoming to women. A striking example is Dr. James Barry, who attended Edinburgh Medical School and served as a British Army surgeon. Barry performed one of the first successful cesarean sections in the world, but it was only after death that Barry was

A. M. Mesiti (✉)
Department of Surgery, Weill Cornell Medicine, New York Presbyterian Hospital,
New York, NY, USA
e-mail: anm9360@nyp.org

H. L. Yeo
Associate Professor of Surgery, Weill Medical College of Cornell University,
New York, NY, USA
e-mail: hey9002@med.cornell.edu

K. Yoon-Flannery et al. (eds.), *Women in Surgery*,
https://doi.org/10.1007/978-3-032-10971-2_3

discovered to be a woman who had lived as a man for 56 years in order to be able to practice medicine [3].

Dr. Elizabeth Blackwell and Dr. Emily Jennings Stowe were the first women physicians in the United States and Canada, respectively. Both faced overwhelming discrimination and repeated rejections from medical schools and residency programs. Dr. Blackwell graduated with honors from Geneva Medical College in 1849 and later founded the New York Infirmary for Women and Children and the Women's Medical College of New York. Dr. Stowe graduated from the New York Medical College for Women in 1867 but was not granted a Canadian medical license until 13 years later [11].

Dr. Mary Edwards Walker, the first female surgeon in the US Army, graduated as the second woman from a US medical school [11]. She was awarded the Congressional Medal of Honor in 1865, which was later revoked in 1917. Walker refused to return the medal, and it was reinstated by President Carter decades later [1].

These pioneers paved the way for modern female surgeons. Their sacrifices are best captured by Dr. Marie Mergler, dean of the Women's Hospital Medical College, who said:"No woman studying medicine today will ever know how much it has cost the individuals personally concerned in bringing about these changes… it meant the failure or success of a grand cause." [11]

Advocacy and Representation

Thanks to these pioneers, the representation of women in medicine has improved significantly. Women now make up approximately 50% of medical students in the USA—a milestone reached over the past decade. In surgery, the 2023–2024 AAMC report shows that 49.3% of general surgery residents identify as women [9].

Despite these gains, challenges remain. Women residents experience higher attrition rates than their male counterparts [12]. Intersectional faculty—those underrepresented in medicine—face lower rates of promotion and retention, and intersectional residents have the highest rates of attrition in general surgery [4, 6]. These disparities highlight the need for targeted interventions to promote and retain women in surgery. So, we have learned that there is still work to be done.

Professional organizations such as the American College of Surgeons Women in Surgery Committee (ACS WISC), the Association of Women Surgeons (AWS), and the American Surgical Association have recognized the need to support women surgeons and the unique challenges they face and have built resources and a community for women to come together. These groups have played a vital role in advocating for equity, mentorship, and visibility. These organizations have supported policies around pay parity, equity, and child and family planning, helping to equalize the profession.

Cultural Change and Family Planning

The evolution of surgical culture has been slow, but deliberate and focused efforts, such as those by professional societies and individual researchers, have made a difference. From revising training structures to accommodate family life to implementing policies that address harassment and bias, institutions have begun to recognize that diversity strengthens the profession.

Still, the past teaches us that change does not happen passively. It requires active leadership, intentional change, and persistence. The voices of women must be heard not only in conversations about equity, but also in decisions that shape the future of surgical education and practice.

The path to becoming a surgeon is long and demanding, often overlapping with a woman's childbearing years. Historically, many women surgeons delayed or forewent having children due to cultural expectations and the lack of institutional support. Some were even asked if they planned to drop out upon becoming pregnant.

Recent studies have shown that female surgeons face increased risks of pregnancy complications, including spontaneous abortion, preterm delivery, fetal growth restriction, and congenital malformations. They are also more likely to experience infertility and require reproductive assistance. Pregnancy loss rates among female surgeons are double that of the general population [7].

These findings have led to increased awareness and policy changes. In 2021, the American Board of Surgery revised its parental leave policy to offer protected and compensated leave for trainees [2]. Institutions like the University of Michigan and the University of Wisconsin have implemented lactation support programs [5]. The American College of Surgeons has issued comprehensive guidelines supporting parental leave and lactation for practicing surgeons [10]. A recent JAMA Surgery article also called for policies to support residents experiencing pregnancy loss [8]. However, there is still much work to be done.

Conclusion

The field of surgery has evolved significantly, thanks to the resilience and determination of early women physicians and surgeons. Their legacy continues to inspire and guide efforts to improve diversity, equity, and support for women in surgery. While progress has been made, ongoing advocacy and structural change are essential to ensure that future generations of women surgeons can thrive—both professionally and personally.

References

1. Ferry G. Mary Edwards Walker: military surgeon who wore the trousers. Lancet. 2020;395(10220):263.
2. General Surgery Resident Leave Policy | ABS. https://www.absurgery.org/resources/abs-policies/policy-leave/. Accessed January 12, 2025.
3. Hurwitz B, Richardson R. Inspector General James Barry MD: putting the woman in her place. BMJ. 1989;298(6669):299–305.
4. Johnson J, Mesiti A, Brouwer J, Shui AM, Sosa JA, Yeo HL. Surgeon intersectionality and academic promotion and retention in the US. JAMA Surg. 2024;159(4):383–388.
5. Livingston-Rosanoff D, Shubeck SP, Kanters AE, et al. Got milk? design and implementation of a lactation support program for surgeons. Ann Surg. 2019;270(1):31–32.
6. Mesiti A, Johnson J, Brouwer J, Shui AM, Yeo H, Sosa JA. The Effect of Intersectionality on Attrition among US General Surgery Trainees. Ann Surg. 2024.
7. Rangel EL, Castillo-Angeles M, Easter SR, et al. Incidence of infertility and pregnancy complications in US female surgeons. JAMA Surg. 2021;156(10):905–915.
8. Siderides C, Cain-Trivette CJ, Garrett KA. Addressing Pregnancy Loss in Surgical Residency-A Call for Policy Protection. JAMA Surg. 2025.
9. Table B3. Number of Active Residents, by Type of Medical School, GME Specialty, and Gender | AAMC. https://www.aamc.org/data-reports/students-residents/data/report-residents/2023/table-b3-number-active-residents-type-medical-school-gme-specialty-and-gender. Accessed May 4, 2024.
10. The American College of Surgeons. Revised Statement on the Importance of Workplace Support for Pregnancy, Parental Leave, and Lactation for Practicing Surgeons. https://www.facs.org/about-acs/statements/revised-statement-on-the-importance-of-workplace-support-for-pregnancy-parental-leave-and-lactation-for-practicing-surgeons/. Accessed May 14, 2024.
11. Wirtzfeld DA. The history of women in surgery. Can J Surg. 2009;52(4):317–320.
12. Yeo HL, Abelson JS, Symer MM, et al. Association of time to attrition in surgical residency with individual resident and programmatic factors. JAMA Surg. 2018;153(6):511–517.

Part II
The Decision to Pursue a Surgical Career

Chapter 4
Motivations and Inspirations

Maureen D. Moore

Introduction

Elizabeth Blackwell is credited with being the first woman admitted to medical school in the mid-1800s [1]. Prior to that, women were banned from practicing medicine. Fast forward to 2025, and the number of women entering practice not only in medicine but also in surgery has exponentially increased [1]. The number of women in leadership positions is on the rise, affording representation of inspirational leadership [1]. Despite this increase in female surgical leadership, there remains an underrepresentation [1, 2]. With this, it is important to explore what drives women to enter and stay in surgery, allowing them to be leaders in their field.

Personal Motivations

There are numerous personal motivations that can inspire women to pursue a surgical career. One motivation that is discussed often among female surgeons is a deep passion for precision and problem-solving. More specifically, the intellectual draw of surgery necessitates complex decision-making, anatomy, and hands-on work. Additionally, many women interested in surgery find that seeing "immediate" and "tangible" results after a surgical operation brings instant gratification. Moreover, many are motivated by overcoming personal or societal challenges and proving their capabilities—resilience in the face of doubt.

M. D. Moore (✉)
Assistant Professor of Surgery, Department of Surgery, Cooper University Hospital,
Cooper Medical School of Rowan University, Camden, NJ, USA
e-mail: moore-maureen@cooperhealth.edu

K. Yoon-Flannery et al. (eds.), *Women in Surgery*,
https://doi.org/10.1007/978-3-032-10971-2_4

Role Models and Mentors

On a personal note, I was inspired to pursue a career in medicine at a young age by watching my father, John M. Daly, M.D., a surgical oncologist, treat countless patients. I was afforded the luxury of "weekend rounds with Dad," where I watched him sit on the patient's bed, calm their fears and worries, discuss surgical or post-surgical plans, and finally give them a compassionate wiggle of their toe before leaving the room. His approach to medicine was deeply rooted in empathy, precision, and an unwavering commitment to his patients' dignity and hope. I watched him not only perform complex surgeries with exceptional skill but also sit beside patients and families with quiet strength and understanding during their most vulnerable moments. He was a surgeon-scientist—a true "triple threat." His vision of care—where science and compassion walk hand in hand—continues to guide and inspire my own path in medicine.

At age 11, my mother, a nurse, was diagnosed with appendiceal adenocarcinoma. Throughout her multiple surgeries, chemotherapy and radiation treatments, CT scans—I was with her. Watching her confront cancer with courage, grace, and strength deeply shaped my understanding of medicine and the human spirit. She had an inspirational quote that we both were quite fond of that is now inscribed on her mass card from her funeral—"Courage does not always roar, sometimes it's the quiet voice at the end of the day saying 'I will try again tomorrow'."

Needless to say, my parents served as role models and mentors for me throughout my early journey through medicine and surgery. Unfortunately, both of my parents have since passed, but the lessons they taught me continue to be my guiding light. Now, many of you may not have situations such as mine where a family member or friend has influenced your career choice. You may, however, have had a professor, an attending, or a laboratory director who has served as a role model or mentor for your surgical career. If neither of those is true—seek out mentorship and guidance—the path of a surgeon is molded together, with mentors to guide.

Defining Moments

For some, the decision to pursue surgery is sparked by a single transformative moment—that "Aha moment;" for others, it is the result of a series of meaningful experiences that, over time, make a surgical career feel both natural and inevitable. Some surgeons remember a pivotal procedure—whether successful or not—that ultimately affirmed their path toward a career in surgery. Inspiration to follow the surgical profession may have come through the guidance of a mentor or a personal experience within the surgical realm. Whichever the case may be, I urge you to keep those defining moments in your pocket and on those tough days—recollect them—remember your why, your reason, and keep pushing forward.

Conclusion

The emotional landscape of a surgical career is broad—fear, exhilaration, doubt, and triumph. Personal motivations, role models/mentors, and defining moments will help steady the variable emotions and allow you to thrive as a woman in surgery.

Keywords
Surgical career, inspirations, motivation

References

1. Pories, S.E., et al., *Leadership in American Surgery: Women are Rising to the Top.* Ann Surg, 2019. **269**(2): p. 199–205.
2. Abelson, J.S., et al., *The climb to break the glass ceiling in surgery: trends in women progressing from medical school to surgical training and academic leadership from 1994 to 2015.* Am J Surg, 2016. **212**(4): p. 566–572 e1.

Chapter 5
Overcoming Challenges and Hurdles

Jennifer F. Tseng

> *I told [Samuel Johnson] I had been that morning at a meeting of the people called Quakers, where I had heard a woman preach. Johnson: "Sir, a woman's preaching is like a dog's walking on his hind legs. It is not done well; but you are surprised to find it done at all."*
>
> James Boswell: Life of Samuel Johnson (1791)

Surgeons succeed. By definition, to become a surgeon is to have worked hard, passed the tests with flying colors, and survived rigorous training. In practice, surgeons make life-or-death decisions every day, are the acknowledged leaders of their teams, and perform extraordinary feats for complex patients at their most vulnerable.

Women are essential. Females are vital in every sphere of human life—economic, social, political, and cultural. Women make up half the population, bear all offspring, provide the majority of care for the young (and not young), and are a critical part of the paid labor force worldwide, especially in healthcare, education, and agriculture [1].

The dual roles of *surgeon* and *woman* bring a profound and awesome weight to bear on female surgeons. With great importance comes great responsibility, and thus enormous stress from the outside world, and most acutely, from ourselves.

For this chapter, I dove for pearls from my recollections of my journey from undergraduate to Chief and Chair and beyond, as summarized in the six "Tseng

J. F. Tseng (✉)
Professor of Surgery Emerita, Boston University, Boston, MA, USA

Clinical Professor of Surgery, Creighton University, Omaha, NE, USA
e-mail: jennifer.tseng@mac.com

K. Yoon-Flannery et al. (eds.), *Women in Surgery*,
https://doi.org/10.1007/978-3-032-10971-2_5

Tips." Because this chapter is one of many, I will focus this discussion on the challenges and barriers during college, medical school, and surgical training.

Tseng's Tips:
Follow your **gut**.

You're **good enough**.
Just **do your best**, at the time.
Give yourself some **grace**.
Remember your **core values**.
Get **outside** yourself.

Follow your **gut**, cancel the noise.

Women who choose surgery still receive mixed messages from people around them, some of whom may have unacknowledged issues of their own. My advice: to seek input, to earnestly listen to a wide variety of individuals, to thoughtfully consider their advice, but not to value any one person or group of people's advice over your own instincts.

In college, while I had wanted to be a doctor since childhood, I ended up fully exploring the liberal arts, ultimately earning degrees in English (with a feminist studies focus) as well as in Biological Sciences. I still identify as an English major to this day. I wrote earnest papers for erudite Jane Austen scholars, published confessional poetry, and entertained the idea of writing fiction as a career. I was inspired by meeting luminaries like Audre Lorde and Ursula K. Le Guin, and labored on my honors thesis on two mid-career Asian-American women poets. With a lot of angst, including great advice from a fiction professor who advised me to "live life; only then you will have something to write about," I decided to apply to medical school.

My English Chair was shocked. The Stanford Chair of English was an Oxfordian Brit named J. Martin Evans, who, when I broke the bad medical news to him at our English Honors Celebration near graduation, intoned, "My dear girl, you will be wasted as a doctor. When I want a surgeon, I want someone who is cold: a machine, a robot. I don't want someone with finer sensibilities. I still remember that junior essay you wrote on Virginia Woolf; I completely disagreed with your tenets, but you have real talent. The two best places for you to pursue your doctorate in literature would be either the University of Chicago, or Yale …" With some alarm, I scheduled an urgent meeting with my thesis advisor, the poet Adrienne Rich. Adrienne, as opposed to Professor Evans, was thankfully encouraging. I told her I hoped to attend the University of California Medical School in San Francisco, and she said, "Great choice! UCSF reminds me of the 'red brick' universities in England, as opposed to the Oxfords and Cambridges." Adrienne then told me that her physician father had been at Johns Hopkins for his whole career, eventually serving as Chair of Pathology [2]. Adrienne also told me that she had had no female role models or teachers throughout her elite university days learning the canon and striving to be a poet, and that she thought we needed more women in medicine and other less welcoming worlds, "especially in the inner sanctums."

I was familiar with Adrienne Rich's hagiography, including her attending Radcliffe and Oxford and marrying a male Harvard professor she had met as an undergraduate, "because it was expected," before winning the Yale Younger Poets Prize, having major life and cultural changes, and leaving her indelible mark on literature [3]. But what Adrienne so kindly shared about herself with me, an unimportant undergraduate, validated what I really wanted to do. What I heard from Professor Rich was, "This is worthwhile work; it is not my path, but it has value. I support your choices." I try to channel that generosity with others to this day.

I did attend medical school, and it was the right choice. However, I certainly did not plan on surgery. Like many others, I became unexpectedly entranced with surgery during my third year clerkship, and even more attracted during my sub-internship (during May of my third year) at San Francisco General Hospital. It wasn't really the technical aspect in the OR; I could barely see anything while holding the retractors, "waterskiing with [Dr. Larry] Way" or peering between larger males at the table, although watching Nancy Ascher tie knots during a liver transplant (immediately postpartum, having been kicked out of the hospital nursery by the NICU nurses, she gave Dr John Roberts a break) was mesmerizing. What transfixed me was the intensity of the interaction with the patients, and the ability to meet humans, work them up, come up with a plan to help them, execute the plan, and receive short-term feedback as to whether the plan worked, all in real time. The teamwork and the camaraderie were addictive. The pace of the surgical day kept me interested and engaged (when sitting for too long a period of time, I become either irritable or drowsy). And the surgery chief residents seemed to be the most complete doctors in the hospital. They could read an ECG, blood gas, or X-ray; run a code; resuscitate a patient; operate skillfully; and then have sensitive and thoughtful conversations with patients and family about cancer or lethal injuries. Surgeons, like the proto-masculine bullfighters that Hemingway's Jake Barnes idolizes in *The Sun Also Rises,* "live their lives all the way up."

By my last year of medical school, choosing a specialty stumped me. Because of my background and commitment to health equity, OB-GYN was the *a priori* front-runner. I had committed to a year-long Howard Hughes fellowship in endometriosis research before even completing core surgery or medicine. I spent the whole year in the lab, simultaneously entranced with scientific investigation and feeling increasingly guilty that I was more interested in surgery and was also strongly considering internal medicine, potentially primary care, women's health, or medical oncology. In my last year, I did three additional sub-internships, July–September, in medicine, OB, and surgery; I ruled out OB, but could not choose between medicine and surgery. This was during the ancient pre-ERAS period; I actually sent away for hard-copy applications in both internal medicine and surgery. These twin towers of paper sat accusingly on either side of my typewriter on the floor of my room in the Haight-Ashbury that was unfurnished except for a futon mattress and boxes of books. "What do I do?" I asked Molly Cooke, my advisor, who is a brilliant primary care doctor and superb educator who ran our Introduction to Clinical Medicine and was one of the early advocates for AIDS patients in San Francisco. Like Adrienne, Dr. Cooke listened to me and told me her story, which was that she was tapped by legendary Stanford cardiac surgical pioneer Dr. Norman Shumway to be his first female cardiac surgery trainee, but that Dr. Shumway recommended she do a medicine internship first to learn physiology. Molly then fell in love with internal medicine and changed her path. She said, "But I have a fairly similar lifestyle than I would have had in surgery, give or take. I am incredibly busy. I am married to an academic physician, we have two kids, we have crazy lives, we juggle the best we can. Your lifestyle in the end will depend more on YOU than on what specialty you choose. So, choose the path which seems the most fun. You can always change." With that advice, the choice for surgery was crystal clear.

I have *never* regretted the decision to pursue surgery.

For space reasons, I will limit my comments regarding the remaining Tseng's Tips to two anecdotes that bookend my training. First,

You're **good enough**.
Just **do your best**, at the time.
Give yourself some **grace**.

I was born, raised, and educated in the San Francisco Bay Area. In 1995, after I chose the pile of paper less traveled by and applied to surgery, I upended my life to start as a surgery intern across the country at Massachusetts General Hospital in Boston. At MGH, I was in the first intern class that had four female categorical residents out of eight ("*fifty percent*," everyone kept saying, as if this was difficult math), and everyone was agog if not apoplectic. (What had happened to the MGH! What was happening to surgery!) I am not sure any class before us had even three; recent cohorts had zero, one, or at most two. This picture (Fig. 1) with mug shots was tacked up at every nursing station. The four categorical male interns in 1995 were Drs. Hutter, Jackson, Lee, and Tolis. Note how they (with the non-general surgery-categorical interns of any gender) are in alphabetical order; none of us, to my knowledge, ever noticed that the residency education staff stacked the four categorical women (Drs. Saunders [now Walsh], Schwarze, Sims, and Tseng at the end, through mischief or just amazement.) I had a tremendous sense of not belonging and not being good enough all through residency, which started on match day and was not improved by the fact that I was intimidated by all my fellow interns, including one who was born at MGH and continuously raised at Harvard and whose father was a revered cardiologist at the institution to boot, and another one whose direct ancestor founded the hospital (and a family member from a less-favored branch adorned the $20 bill.) I made it through residency with hard work, luck and pluck, an oppressive fear of failure, and unexpected alliances, including with the scrub techs; the OR, floor, and clinic nurses; Karen, the residency office lady; John, the radiology clerk; and Steve, the AV guy. That intern who had his family name on a building became a lifelong friend, and his parents are my honorary godparents. The three "Tseng's tips" above came those times, which must have had some bad in them (which makes for wild & crazy stories but carries no pain today), but I truly remember them as some of the best times of my life.

Finally, one final anecdote at the very end of my training to bookend the first and highlight the last two "Tseng's Tips."

Remember your **core values**.
Get **outside** yourself.

In all, I spent 10 years in residency, lab, and fellowship. I fought many battles, especially with my own doubts during those years, and still had extraordinary fun while doing so. I capped off my training with a 2-year surgical oncology fellowship at the University of Texas M.D. Anderson Cancer Center in Houston; my husband remained in Boston for his academic job. We delayed starting our family during my training because of his unassailable belief that our child would not survive with him as the primary parent while I returned to surgical training. "I would have to call Child Protective Services on myself" is a direct quote from him. Moving to Texas, I became close with the men—they were all men—with whom I finished my fellowship, and we are friends to this day. They happen to all be married to women who came with them to Houston. My co-fellows had all already been blessed with children. They had also been blessed with their amazing wives, who are great women; two of them were physicians, and one was a nurse I had known since my internship. We were insanely busy in the hospital, but my co-fellows' wives would organize terrific parties and warm social functions; I always had a great time and learned a lot about hosting and making everyone feel comfortable, something I still carry with me to this day. Fellowship was amazing, if somewhat truncated because my "research time" in the first half of my second and final year was spent spending 6 months as the "Super Chief" back in Boston instead of doing relaxing research. Amazingly, ostensibly living in the same apartment as your spouse but him only seeing your dirty scrubs pile up in the hamper (because you are the attending on-call 24/7 for 6 months straight for acute and non-designated elective general, thoracic, and vascular surgeries, plus on-call in-house every fourth 24 h for Level 1 Trauma, and are also the daytime elective attending for two active ORs M-F) is more stressful to a marriage than being in different parts of the country. After finishing this trying Super-Chief time and my returning to Houston, somewhat miraculously, my husband and I became pregnant "as soon as we were not actively trying NOT to" in February of my last year of training! Because this was the Dark Ages of Pregnancy Shame, I only told the good news to my Program Director and my Chair; I had my prenatal visits on my vacation in Boston; any local appointments were done *ad hoc* and on the down-low, which I have addressed elsewhere [4]. (I would make different choices today and have so advised many younger people of different genders.)

Finale

Drumroll: cut to graduation from surgical oncology fellowship! My husband flew in for the graduation dinner and to help move me and my stuff back to our newly acquired suburban house and to my pending job at UMass Worcester. I was so excited to finally have my partner at my side and looked forward to us finally sharing the graduation experience with my fellow fellows and their spouses as a couple.

When it was time for dinner, which was open seating, I had a nasty shock. It turned out the other five graduating fellows and their wives had seats for themselves at one table, with no room for my husband and me. I was taken aback, saddened, and felt suddenly, once again, like I was not a member of the club, no matter how hard I tried. I do not believe I created any kind of a scene, but I *may* have spent some time in a bathroom stall crying quietly. (One could blame being hormonal, but "hormones" have never seemed to bother me on any other occasion, pregnant or otherwise).

I emerged from the bathroom. I found my coffee-comrade fellow Keith Delman had, in the meantime, tried to get the staff to allow two more seats to be added to the table, but they were really meant for 8 and would absolutely *not* accommodate 12. In the end, my husband and I had an amazing dinner seated with some of the first-year fellows, including Waddah Al-Refaie, now my research brother and ally of many years. Everyone survived and thrived. I have only one picture for the day, and that is the image I choose to remember. For the after-dinner photo, the fellowship organized the trainees and the faculty in a tableau that shows the graduating 2- and 3-year general surgical oncology fellows (with the two 1-year breast fellows joining us) all beaming in the front row.

Between the quality time spent in the restaurant bathroom and more time later while packing up a slew of IKEA furniture in the Houston heat, a few things became clear to me: No one meant ill. We're all the center of our own universes. I never thought to pre-plan where we would sit at dinner. I never discussed with anyone ahead of time or during the cocktail hour or tried to "save seats," and why would my spouse think to do so? The other graduating fellows were seated together because their wives organized it. These couples that had formed long-lasting couple- and family-based bonds over several years were to be separated from each other, and wanted to have one last hurrah together. It doesn't mean they didn't like me. (Or as other, more cynical people might say, "Even if they don't, so what? ") One could just as easily blame the restaurant, the dinner organizers, or, of course, the spouse. (Or hormones! Husbands and hormones are always safe scapegoats.) But what benefit accrues from casting blame on anything or anyone, including oneself? Zero, unless learning and evolution occur. What mattered to me—my core values—were the reasons why I made the choices I did, which had led me to that moment, graduating from surgical oncology fellowship, having survived a commuting relationship with a superstar academic spouse, and embarking on a position that would both allow us to start our family together and to empower me to begin my chosen career in surgery.

Conclusions

Challenges exist in choosing and pursuing surgery, especially for women and those not traditionally seen as surgeons. While barriers exist, and the playing field is not level, I propose that it is very much worth it for women, for the field of surgery, and for patients and trainees, for us to join the game.

References

1. UN Women: For All Women and Girls. https://www.unwomen.org/en
2. Arnold Rice Rich. https://en.wikipedia.org/wiki/Arnold_Rice_Rich
3. Adrienne Rich. https://en.wikipedia.org/wiki/Adrienne_Rich
4. Tseng JF. 2023 A. Hamblin Letton Lecture. *The American Surgeon™*. 2023;89(7):3029–3036. https://doi.org/10.1177/00031348231188796 https://journals.sagepub.com/doi/10.1177/00031348231188796

Chapter 6
Educational and Training Considerations

Rebekah Huckeby, Haley Eversman, Madolyn Conant, Audrey R. Yang, and Tanya Anand

It was the end of my first day on a new rotation. As a third-year medical student, I had spent the last few months going from rotation to rotation in a cycle of new residents and attendings. I felt a wave of dread wash over me as the words started to tumble out of my attending's mouth, "So what specialty do you think you want to go into?" he asked intently. The residents in the group curiously looked up from their notes. I was faced with a decision between honesty and reservation. Do I tell the truth, or do I give a vague answer such as, "I am just keeping my options open at the moment?" I chose authenticity and replied, "I am really interested in trauma surgery." I felt all eyes on me in that moment, with looks varying from confusion to surprise, and I heard him say, "You? Trauma surgery? You are way too nice to be going into surgery, let alone trauma surgery! Just promise me that you won't let them change you." I was slightly taken aback by the sentiment, but unfortunately, I was not a stranger to this type of reaction. I had gotten it many times before from other attendings and residents. Mostly, I had heard comments such as "but what about work-life balance?" or "don't you want to have a family?" or even "don't worry, we still have time to convert you away from surgery." I had always prided myself on being caring and compassionate. I had never thought that these traits would be viewed as an obstacle to becoming a surgeon.

R. Huckeby
Division of Trauma, Surgical Critical Care, Burns and Acute Care Surgery,
Department of Surgery, University of Arizona, Tucson, AZ, USA
e-mail: rfhuckeby@arizona.edu

H. Eversman · M. Conant · A. R. Yang
Department of Surgery, University of Arizona, Tucson, AZ, USA
e-mail: eversman@arizona.edu; mconant@arizona.edu; aryang@arizona.edu

T. Anand (✉)
Clinical Assistant Professor of Surgery, Division of Trauma, Surgical Critical Care, Burns and Acute Care Surgery, Department of Surgery, University of Arizona, Tucson, AZ, USA
e-mail: tanyaanand@surgery.arizona.edu

K. Yoon-Flannery et al. (eds.), *Women in Surgery*,
https://doi.org/10.1007/978-3-032-10971-2_6

As medical students, we are often asked what specialty we would like to go into when we meet a new team member, particularly attendings. At first, this question appears innocent; however, it generates an interesting reaction and subsequently reshapes my clinical experience in the rotation. As another example, I personally noticed a shift in attitude when I would divulge that I wanted to pursue neurosurgery. My treatment proposals began to be viewed differently. They would be considered too aggressive despite following guidelines. Comments such as "I must find general medicine topics boring" despite my repeatedly expressed interest or that I "give off neurosurgery energy" impacted my eagerness to freely participate. As a result, I began to withhold this information to avoid being stereotyped by this negative perception of a female with a "surgical personality." When I expressed that I may be debating psychiatry as I liked the inpatient management complexity, I was told I would not do well there and would be "a tough love psychiatrist" and would be frustrated with patients and be unable to show empathy. This shocked me as psychiatry had been my original goal, and I find myself to be incredibly empathetic and giving.

The comments that were directed towards us were not directed towards our male colleagues. There appeared to be a notion that women must come across as aggressive, possibly more masculine, for others to believe they will succeed in a surgical career or be categorized into a surgical subspecialty. It demonstrates the work still needed to make an equitable and encouraging environment for women who decide to pursue surgery.

"If society will not admit of women's free development, then society must be remodeled." Elizabeth Blackwell spoke these words in the 1800s and played an instrumental role in advocating for female physicians. Her accomplishments allowed women to not only dream, but to achieve. Soon after, Dr. Mary Edwards Walker added to this fire and became the first female surgeon in the United States. The number of female physicians remained low throughout the 1900s until around 1970, when there was a rapid increase from 2% to 24% of physicians being female by 2001 [1]. Recently, it has been noted that only 47.9% of medical student graduates and 45.6% of residents are female despite the majority of applicants being female [2]. Of the women that do become residents, many report not being addressed by their formal title by staff and patients more often than their male colleagues and are not recognized for accomplishments via awards or opportunities as often [3, 4]. Additionally, around one-third of female physicians reported being subjected to biases in their careers [5]. Despite the challenges faced by female physicians, it has been found that their patients have lower mortality rates and shorter lengths of stay in the hospital as compared to their male counterparts when treated by female physicians [6].

The above experiences by female trainees highlight challenges that women face daily in their trek to becoming surgeons. Comments, such as those noted above, may enforce a false notion that a female student requires a "surgical personality" (i.e., assertive, independent, demanding) to become a competent and compassionate surgeon, thus driving away promising candidates in whom the above notion does not align with their own self-perception [7]. As a student's understanding of their own career shapes itself, support and guidance by non-surgeons is equally important to the guidance offered by surgeons. Practical and objective information regarding the demands of their own specialty should be conveyed to the student, such that the trainee can create an accurate picture in their mind of whether their chosen field will fulfill their personal and professional goals. By doing so, there is a high likelihood that the career choice that is made is an adequately informed decision.

With the challenges noted above, there are triumphs as well. For the first time since 2019, a majority of medical students were female. This trend has only continued, with 57% of medical students being female [8]. These increasing numbers are likely secondary to increased mentorship and resources for trainees. Though improving, more female surgeon mentors are needed as they serve as role models for those wanting to understand how to balance career challenges and responsibilities, as well as caregiving concerns [9]. There are numerous resources stemming from surgical societies that provide supportive avenues for women trainees [9, 10]. The Association of Women Surgeons (AWS), The American College of Surgeons (ACS), and The American Association for the Surgery of Trauma (AAST) are just a few organizations that have dedicated resources in the form of social media, committee involvement, speaking opportunities, and much more to provide that supportive environment for networking and career advancement [9, 10].

References

1. Wirtzfeld DA. The history of women in surgery. *Can J Surg*. 2009;52(4):317–320.
2. 2018–2019 The State of Women in Academic Medicine: Exploring Pathways to Equity. AAMC. Accessed May 1, 2025. https://www.aamc.org/data-reports/data/2018-2019-state-women-academic-medicine-exploring-pathways-equity
3. Silver JK, Slocum CS, Bank AM, et al. Where Are the Women? The Underrepresentation of Women Physicians Among Recognition Award Recipients From Medical Specialty Societies. *PMR*. 2017;9(8):804–815. doi:https://doi.org/10.1016/j.pmrj.2017.06.001
4. Files JA, Mayer AP, Ko MG, et al. Speaker Introductions at Internal Medicine Grand Rounds: Forms of Address Reveal Gender Bias. *J Womens Health 2002*. 2017;26(5):413–419. https://doi.org/10.1089/jwh.2016.6044
5. Templeton K, Nilsen KM, Walling A. Issues Faced by Senior Women Physicians: A National Survey. *J Womens Health 2002*. 2020;29(7):980–988. https://doi.org/10.1089/jwh.2019.7910
6. Wallis CJ, Ravi B, Coburn N, Nam RK, Detsky AS, Satkunasivam R. Comparison of postoperative outcomes among patients treated by male and female surgeons: a population based matched cohort study. *BMJ*. 2017;359:j4366. https://doi.org/10.1136/bmj.j4366
7. Fassiotto M, Li J, Maldonado Y, Kothary N. Female Surgeons as Counter Stereotype: The Impact of Gender Perceptions on Trainee Evaluations of Physician Faculty. *J Surg Educ*. 2018;75(5):1140–1148. https://doi.org/10.1016/j.jsurg.2018.01.011
8. Women in medicine make gains, but obstacles remain. AAMC. Accessed May 1, 2025. https://www.aamc.org/news/women-medicine-make-gains-obstacles-remain
9. Oppenheimer-Velez M, Sims C, Labiner H, et al. Women Empowering Women: Assessing the American College of Surgeons Women in Surgery Committee Mentorship Program. *J Am Coll Surg*. 2022;235(2):375. https://doi.org/10.1097/XCS.0000000000000272
10. Luc JGY, Stamp NL, Antonoff MB. Social media in the mentorship and networking of physicians: Important role for women in surgical specialties. *Am J Surg*. 2018;215(4):752–760. https://doi.org/10.1016/j.amjsurg.2018.02.011

Chapter 7
Career Planning and Goal Setting

Mara A. Piltin

Introduction

The best professional advice I have been given is to *act as if you are the level above your current position*. This can be applied to medical training, business, administration, leadership, and many other aspects of life. This concept is similarly summarized in the recommendation to behave like the person you want to become, or as is commonly paraphrased from Ralph Waldo Emerson's poetically abridged perspectives, "That which we persist in doing becomes easier to do—not that the nature of the thing has changed, but that our power to do has increased" [2].

When envisioning a fruitful career and setting future goals, it is important to assume that role in your mind. If it feels simultaneously empowering and uncomfortable to picture yourself there, you are probably on the right track. As a breast and melanoma surgical oncologist who trained in a smaller community hospital setting for osteopathic medical school and residency, I set a career vision for an academic practice at a large institution.

Like many, I have faced uphill battles. From a career perspective, to achieve a position that matched my career goals, I found myself navigating hurdles such as coming from a small training program and the inherent challenges that accompany this. A stigma in the surgical field toward osteopathic training, roadblocks to productive and meaningful research, networking limitations, and others. However, what has remained consistent is confidence in the quality of patient care I provide, my surgical skillset, grit, and self-worth. With an interest in forward progress and academic growth, I used goal-setting to advance my career.

M. A. Piltin (✉)
Vice Chair of Innovation, Department of Surgery, Assistant Professor of Surgery,
Division of Surgical Oncology, Mayo Clinic, Rochester, NY, USA
e-mail: Piltin.Mara@Mayo.edu

K. Yoon-Flannery et al. (eds.), *Women in Surgery*,
https://doi.org/10.1007/978-3-032-10971-2_7

Career planning can seem daunting, especially when beginning your journey in the healthcare profession. There are innumerable measures of success, and the further along in medical training you get, the less linear the concept of success becomes. Initially, most physicians-in-training have similar goals: competitive MCAT scores, acceptance into medical school, high board scores, and matching a top residency/fellowship choice. Once you have ticked the boxes and ventured into designing your career, the pathways become boundless, and the ability to model yourself like those who came before you less clear.

Studies have shown that the act of writing down career goals makes them more concrete and achievable. Individuals who write their goals and/or engage in goal-setting exercises are significantly more likely to achieve success [1, 3, 4]. Additionally, it has been shown that there appears to be a higher success rate in goal achievement for individuals who share their goals with friends and family than those who internalize them [1]. Coined in 1981, the SMART technique is commonly referenced and offers a practical framework to organize one's aims. It is an acronym for Specific, Measurable, Assignable, Realistic, and Time-related, and although originally described for management level, it can certainly be adapted for personal career growth [5].

I will share a few more subjective principles that have helped guide me:

Remain True to Yourself Despite Personal Evolution It is my opinion that growth and change are necessary to continue evolving professionally and personally. However, there is great value in reflecting on what aspects of yourself you like, respect, and value. Uphold those facets through change, but acknowledge that the aspects that fit those criteria may fluctuate. Allowing for preservation of those components as you manage your professional career will give you great pride.

Find Good Mentors Naturally Throughout the course of medical training, mentorship programs will exist and may link you with excellent advisors, colleagues, and friends. More commonly, though, established programs that match individuals with a mentor lack the natural magnetism that makes a great mentor-mentee relationship. Whether you engage in mentorship programs or not, find individuals who challenge you, offer insight, and most importantly are willing to make time for you. Often these are the individuals whom you goal set and career mimic the most because you admire them, or aspects of them.

Become a Good Mentor By allowing yourself to mentor others, this will force you to identify the components of mentorship that you value and seek [6]. This is a form of self-reflection because it will help you identify your own successes and failures to guide and inform those coming after you. This is an excellent way to highlight your own career strengths and weaknesses while simultaneously assisting the next generation of providers.

First, Be a "Yes Woman"...

...Then only accept what you enjoy. Early in your career, you may discover components of your work such as academia, leadership, global outreach, authorship, innovation, science, education, or others that you did not know you had a passion for due to a lack of exposure or different perspectives. For example, data entry as a medical student is not the same as involvement in a funded research group that collaborates across disciplines, and saying no to the umbrella of research because of an early experience may close the door on wonderful opportunities. Use the beginning phase of your career to absorb what you can from a multitude of experiences. Soon, you will start to detect a layering of what you enjoy versus what feels like work, leading to clarity and confidence in the opportunities and offers you decline.

Celebrate Your Successes Women have historically undervalued their worth, with numerous studies identifying a significant wage gap, including modern reports revealing that women physicians and surgeons are compensated 71% of their male counterparts. This discrepancy remains true when adjusting for specialty, geography, work hours, and other potential confounders [7]. A survey-based study revealed that female general surgery residents had lower salary expectations and were less likely to negotiate their starting salary after residency [8]. Do not be afraid to ask for more, apply for the leadership position, self-promote, or take a seat at the table. Design your career and set goals based on what matters to you, and allow yourself to celebrate your wins and highlight your successes. High self-esteem has been shown to correlate with career success and the achievement of value-aligned and meaningful pursuits [9].

As a female surgeon, there is one additional consideration I urge you to reflect on as you think about goal setting. Have a family if you want to, don't if you don't. Avoid letting fears of career disruption get in the way of building a meaningful and fulfilling life outside of work, however that looks for you.

Conclusion

While I remain early in my career, I have learned a lot about how to manage opportunities and challenges. Surgery is a historically male-dominated profession with high stress and high demand which can often feel daunting to take on as a woman, especially as a young woman. Setting goals, maintaining persistence, pushing oneself beyond their comfort zone, trusting their strengths, and seeking support from successful mentors and colleagues will serve you well.

References

1. Matthews, G. (2015, May). *The impact of commitment, accountability, and written goals on goal achievement.* Paper presented at the Ninth Annual International Conference of the Psychology Research Unit, Athens Institute for Education and Research, Athens, Greece
2. Emerson, R. W. (1860). *Power.* In *The conduct of life.* Ticknor and Fields.
3. Morisano, D., Hirsh, J. B., Peterson, J. B., Pihl, R. O., & Shore, B. M. (2010). Setting, elaborating, and reflecting on personal goals improves academic performance. *Journal of Applied Psychology, 95*(2), 255–264.
4. Gollwitzer, P. M., & Sheeran, P. (2006). Implementation intentions and goal achievement: A meta-analysis. *Advances in Experimental Social Psychology, 38*, 69–119.
5. Doran, G. T. (1981, November). There's a S.M.A.R.T. way to write management's goals and objectives. *Management Review, 70*(11), 35–36.
6. Sadowski, E. B., & Schrager, S. (2016). Achieving career satisfaction: Personal goal setting and prioritizing for the clinician educator. *Journal of Graduate Medical Education, 8*(4), 494–497.
7. Asgari, M. M., Carr, P. L., & Bates, C. K. (2019). Closing the gender wage gap and achieving professional equity in medicine. *JAMA, 321*(17), 1665–1666.
8. Grey, A. D., Williams, A. M., Killelea, B. K., Chagpar, A. B., & Tossas, O. (2019). Career goals, salary expectations, and salary negotiation among male and female general surgery residents. *JAMA Surgery, 154*(9), 861–868.
9. Judge, T. A., Bono, J. E., Erez, A., & Locke, E. A. (2005). Core self-evaluations and job and life satisfaction: The mediating role of self-concordant goals. *Journal of Applied Psychology, 90*(2), 257–268.

Chapter 8
Mentorship in Surgery

Tatiana Hoyos Gomez and Karen Brasel

Mentorship in surgery is about more than technical skills—it shapes values, character, and leadership, ensuring the profession upholds its standards while adapting to modern challenges. Research highlights its importance in creating a healthier, more resilient workforce, and for women and individuals with intersectional identities, it plays a crucial role in fostering inclusivity and addressing unique challenges in the field [2].

The kind of mentorship someone might need can change depending on where they are in their career and what they prefer. These days, it's less about having one mentor for your entire journey and more about building a "mosaic" of mentors, creating a team of people, each offering something specific—whether it's a skill, perspective, or shared experience. Different types of mentorship can work for different relationships, and they are not mutually exclusive. Here are a few examples.

Traditional mentorship would be a senior surgeon mentoring a junior mentee through career development, clinical practice, and work-life integration. This is a hierarchical model, where the mentor is the primary source of knowledge. Peer mentorship would be two early-career female surgeons, both navigating academic progression and facing similar challenges. They meet to share strategies for overcoming these hurdles and provide each other with emotional support. This kind of mentorship fosters camaraderie and mutual understanding, making it easier for them to communicate openly and address issues that are specific to their shared experiences. The Women in Trauma Surgery and Women in Surgery mentorship

T. Hoyos Gomez (✉)
Oregon Health & Science University, Portland, OR, USA
e-mail: hoyosgom@ohsu.edu

K. Brasel
American Board of Surgery, Philadelphia, PA, USA

Oregon Health & Science University, Portland, OR, USA
e-mail: kbrasel@absurgery.org

K. Yoon-Flannery et al. (eds.), *Women in Surgery*,
https://doi.org/10.1007/978-3-032-10971-2_8

circle is a great example of group mentorship, where a group of female surgeons at various stages of their careers meet regularly with one or more mentors. Each member may offer expertise in different areas, encouraging the exchange of experiences and fostering a sense of community. Members benefit not only from professional guidance but also from sponsorship and networking opportunities. Formal mentorship is a structured program that may include regular scheduled meetings to review academic progress, clinical skills, and career goals. These programs often involve established guidelines for mentor-mentee interactions, such as a minimum number of meetings per year, periodic evaluations, and feedback mechanisms.

The role of professional societies in formal or structured mentorship is important, particularly for those who do not have access to a mentorship program in their own institution or practice. A formal mentorship example within a surgical society is the Association of Women Surgeons (AWS) mentorship program. AWS pairs junior surgeons or residents with senior surgeons in a structured framework. Regular check-ins, goal-setting, and feedback mechanisms are part of the formal structure, ensuring that mentees receive the support they need. Mentorship "pods" or teams are small groups of mentors and mentees with a more collaborative mentorship focus. It might include senior surgeons, junior surgeons, and trainees, and it creates a very dynamic flow where everyone learns from each other, and it benefits from a very rich pool of lived experiences and perspectives. This form of mentorship does particularly well in promoting a sense of community. An example of a mentorship pod could include a junior attending, a fellow, a chief resident, and a junior resident, not only connecting peers in training but also providing insights into early career challenges, building a practice, and overall transition to practice and independence. Informal mentorship in surgery is probably the most common type of mentorship, where a surgeon informally guides a colleague, providing career advice or personal insights on balancing the demands of surgery and family life, based on their own experiences, often in a more casual, spontaneous setting. This dynamic can also be reciprocal, defined as reverse mentorship, with mutual exchange of knowledge and perspectives.

When I reflect on the factors that shaped my journey toward achieving my goals, mentorship stands out as one of the most significant. Over the course of my career, I didn't have a single mentor who met all my needs, but rather a constellation or team of mentors who appeared at the right time, offering guidance in ways that were uniquely suited to each stage of my development. Having the right mentor for the right challenge was instrumental in my success. Equally important was the diversity of my mentors—not just those who shared my identity and aspirations, but also those whose perspectives challenged me to think differently. One particularly meaningful example occurred early in my path to pursuing a surgical residency in the USA as an international medical graduate; the journey was daunting—a steep, uphill climb often met with skepticism and discouragement. Through networking and serendipitous connections, I met a female surgeon who became a pivotal figure in my professional life. She, too, was an international medical graduate from South America, a wife, a mother, and a surgeon. Seeing someone who not only shared my heritage but had also reached the pinnacle of a career I dreamed of gave me a profound sense of possibility. Now, having walked this path myself, I feel a deep responsibility to give back. I mentor medical students and aspiring surgeons whose stories echo my own. It's not just about offering guidance—it's about creating a bridge for those who come after me, just as my mentors did for me.

Mentorship, however, is not a one-way street. In guiding students and residents, I've learned as much from them as they have from me. They've reminded me that there's no singular path to success. Instead, there are countless ways to navigate challenges, make decisions, and thrive. Each relationship, each shared story, enriches my understanding and keeps me grounded in the beauty of growth and mutual learning.

One of my most impactful role models, someone who has always looked for opportunities to sponsor me, my co-author on this chapter shares her experience: "The most important things that I have learned about mentorship are that structure is important, the understanding of the importance of the life-cycle of a mentorship relationship, and the value of mentorship teams that complement each other. The mentorship relationships that I have now benefit from structure. Scheduling routine meetings is the first step, and preparation is the next. The road that a mentee is likely to follow is not going to be my road, and in order to be successful in helping guide someone, I need to understand their goals, knowledge, skills, and commitment.

I had the good fortune of having a mentor who was very instrumental early in my career. It took me longer than it should have to understand that in order to continue growth in my later career, I needed to expand my mentorship team to include those who had skills that neither my early mentor or I had, and could sponsor me to provide other opportunities for my growth."

Despite progress, significant disparities persist in areas such as the gender pay gap, slower academic progression, and limited access to leadership roles. Just to name a few examples, women are hired at lower salaries despite equal qualifications and face an 18% lower likelihood of attaining full professorship compared to men. Leadership roles are similarly male-dominated, with only 15% of surgical chairs and 16% of medical school deanships held by women [1]. To drive progress, the House of Surgery must embrace a cultural shift—one that actively promotes and supports women, while addressing the unique challenges we face. Mentorship and sponsorship serve as critical tools in this transformation. It is up to all of us to embrace these opportunities: to seek guidance, to offer support, and to create networks that uplift and empower women in surgery.

Here Are Some Actionable Insights

Define your goals and categorize your mentorship needs, whether it is professional development, scholarship, work-life integration, leadership development, education, or technical skills.

Be Proactive and Take Initiative Don't wait for mentorship to come to you, or for your institution to propose a mentorship plan, since many don't have one; advocate for yourself by seeking it.

Diversify Your Mentorship Network Try to have a mentor within your specialty, within your institution, and outside your institution for diversity of perspective.

Be Specific and Intentional Schedule regular meetings. When meeting your mentor, come prepared with well-thought-out, specific questions. This demonstrates that you value your mentor's time and helps ensure the conversation remains focused and productive.

Join Professional Societies Become a member of professional societies relevant to your professional, academic, or nonacademic and personal interests and participate in committees in those societies. If a society doesn't seem to fit, don't get discouraged and try another.

Reciprocate and Engage Always remember that mentorship is a two-way relationship. Show gratitude, provide updates on your progress, and look for ways to support your mentor's work or initiatives.

References

1. Fox, N., Schroll, R., Quiodettis, M., Ito, K., & Bulger, E. M. (2024). Women in trauma surgery: advancing our profession through international collaboration. *Trauma Surg Acute Care Open, 9*(1), e001366. doi:https://doi.org/10.1136/tsaco-2024-001366
2. Gaeta, E. D., Gilbert, M., Johns, A., Jurkovich, G. J., & Wieck, M. M. (2024). Effects of Mentorship on Surgery Residents' Burnout and Well-Being: A Scoping Review. *J Surg Educ, 81*(11), 1592–1601. doi:https://doi.org/10.1016/j.jsurg.2024.08.001

Part III
Training and Education in Surgery

Chapter 9
Fellowship Training

Erika B. Lindholm

Many medical students, when comparing different career paths in medical school, find the option of a 5-year surgical residency daunting, especially when other residency programs have a 3-year commitment. Committing to even more additional years of fellowship is even more daunting before having started any training. Once the years of general surgery residency start to pass, though, and the initial fear is replaced with the understanding of the complexity of what you are learning, the thought of adding time is often welcomed, especially if you are passionate about a field that demands additional years. Beyond the additional time and your passion to pursue your dream career, there are a few key considerations.

At the outset, you need to consider all your options at an early point in your career to put yourself in a position to succeed. For example, even if you start general surgery residency with the intention of being a general surgeon, you should strive to perform well on the Absite and participate in research projects to add to your curriculum vitae, as your goals may change. Preparing for the Absite annually will help you pass your boards at a minimum and, at best, will allow you to pursue a competitive fellowship should you change your mind. Similarly, participating in research projects that result in publication will help in your future pursuit of academic promotion once settled in your career, even if you do not apply for a fellowship. The key point is that following these simple rules will position you for success, even if your career aspirations change over time.

It is axiomatic that career changes are common. Similar to medical students who do not know their future residency, most surgery residents are undecided on what they will pursue after graduation. Part of the process of figuring out your career aspirations is determining what options exist. The best resources are always others

E. B. Lindholm (✉)
Assistant Professor of Pediatrics and Surgery, Division of Pediatric Surgery,
Cooper University Hospital, Cooper Medical School of Rowan University, Camden, NJ, USA
e-mail: lindholm-erika@cooperhealth.edu

K. Yoon-Flannery et al. (eds.), *Women in Surgery*,
https://doi.org/10.1007/978-3-032-10971-2_9

who have been in this situation (or are still in this situation). You should find mentors in specialties that you are interested in, or that have achieved careers via alternative paths. Even internet searches on your dream jobs can be helpful to know what your options are for the future. For example, if you are interested in global surgery, extensive online research will keep you informed on the funded fellowship opportunities that exist. There are so many paths for your career to take, but you need to tailor it according to your goals and interests. Following the "cookbook" formula of the residents that have come before you may not be to your advantage. Similarly, my personal career path changed from surgical oncology to pediatric surgery after completing a pediatric surgical oncology fellowship between my fourth and fifth year of residency. Options exist; you just need to find them.

The above is emblematic of what occurs in your career: as you proceed, you will seek additional time-consuming training opportunities that strengthen your application for competitive fellowships with low match rates. Consequently, pursuing a 2-year fellowship can require an additional 2 years of research time to qualify for that fellowship. Time adds up quickly, and the additional research time does not guarantee you acceptance into any fellowship, a stressful part of the decision-making process when pursuing your passion. As there is no guarantee of matching, I suggest choosing your "extra" years that make you a better surgeon, even if you do not match. In my own experience, I chose a pediatric surgical oncology fellowship with the goal of determining whether to pursue pediatric surgery or oncologic surgery. Most importantly, this training would improve my surgical skills and position me for greater success in any surgical specialty I pursue. Pursuing extra training that will make you a better surgeon will always help you in the future.

One other consideration is that you need a strong family or friend support system to pursue additional training. The long hours in the hospital, combined with difficult call nights and weekends, can strain a partner or spouse, who you will rely on for support and to support your family, should you have one. It is imperative that they are part of the decision-making process, understand what is at stake, and understand the benefits. All fellowships have different requirements (even those in the same field) for working hours and call time, so it is important to have a realistic idea of the amount of time you will need to dedicate to mastering your chosen field.

Finally, it can be helpful to understand the job market in the area you would like to live in and how advanced training will change your career outlook. Adding years of training can improve the quality of life compared to those who did not pursue a competitive fellowship. Residency will give you an understanding of the workflow for different specialties and what you can expect during attending life. In addition, you should discuss with mentors what to expect from a typical job in your specialty, as it can vary greatly between hospitals. Different jobs will require shift work, or overnight calls, and you need to know what to expect to make sure that your expectations align with your reality.

Being tied to an area geographically can be difficult, but it can also let you know if your aspirations are realistic. Look into the job market and check to see if there is a demand for your specialty. After spending so much additional time training, you want to ensure that your future plans are realistic. When you match into your fellowship, start inquiring about job opportunities in your desired community. Let people know that you will be looking for a job in a few years and that you intend to practice in this region. Finally, your attendings in residency and fellowship will be called when it comes time for you to get a job; make sure that you show them that you will be a good partner through your work ethic and dedication to patients. The world of specialties is smaller than you can imagine, and everyone knows everyone.

Chapter 10
Work-Life Integration and Well-Being

Lisa M. Reid

Work-life integration is a relatively new term that has appropriately replaced the term work-life balance. The older term suggested that there was a need for equal time for personal responsibilities as well as for those at work, leaving women with an endless struggle to feel like both areas were given sufficient time. This often led to more stress rather than the happy state that the term suggested. The term work-life integration is more inclusive and realistic, as it accounts for finding wholeness in our personal and professional lives while being accomplished in both arenas.

Work-life integration has been particularly difficult for female surgeons as they face unique pressures in a traditionally male-dominated field. Being a surgeon is challenging due to the rigors of surgical training with long and unpredictable hours. Even after the completion of training, the clinical responsibilities and associated emotional toll involved with caring for patients can be stressful. It is difficult to separate and let go of these stressors in one's personal lifes, and the distinction between work and personal life often become blurred. It is easier said than done to "leave work at work" when you had a challenging case that day, or know that you have a severely ill patient with a surgical complication or a high potential to develop one.

The ability to fully separate work and personal life is unrealistic, and a more realistic goal is to have a model of work-life integration that involves self-awareness, allowing for flexibility and varying prioritization of work and the responsibilities at home. Rather than striving for complete compartmentalization between work and personal life, developing a pattern that includes the blending of career and personal goals is the basis for work-life integration. This has to be an intentional practice, and seeking out resources to help accomplish this goal is crucial. It does not require losing sight of personal identity.

L. M. Reid (✉)
Section of Endocrine Surgery, Cooper University Hospital, Camden, NJ, USA
e-mail: reid-lisa@cooperhealth.edu

K. Yoon-Flannery et al. (eds.), *Women in Surgery*,
https://doi.org/10.1007/978-3-032-10971-2_10

Mentors are crucial as they not only give advice but will also share their own personal experiences. There is an increasing offering of formal mentorship programs in national surgical societies that are available to both trainees and practicing physicians.

Additionally, there are peer support networks and institutional wellness programs that are becoming more common as awareness of the need is apparent. There is data available on the things that can help surgeons attain a healthy view of work-life integration [7]. Two things that should be highlighted are fair compensation and lifestyle changes. While the former is harder to control for, there are strategies that are readily available to all that help foster wellness and prevent burnout. These include the following:

- Getting adequate *sleep*
- Having *hobbies* outside of work
- Daily *exercise*
- Maintaining a healthy *diet*
- Making time to spend with people that matter, as well as time with pets
- Saying *no* to extra work or other commitments that put undue stress on your personal time
- Taking *regular breaks from work*
- Practicing *mindfulness* [8]

One of the consequences of not having work-life integration is burnout. The term was first used in the 1970s by psychotherapist Herbert Freudenberger [1]. The World Health Organization (WHO) defines burnout as an occupational phenomenon and not as a medical diagnosis, though with an ICD-11 definition [2]: "Burnout is a syndrome that results from chronic workplace stress that has not been successfully managed." Other sources such as the Mayo Clinic [3] cite symptoms that are similar to those seen in depression and include the following:

- Exhaustion
- Feeling alienated from work/work activities
- Decrease in performance at work

There has been increasing awareness of the problem of burnout among surgeons, and this is not gender specific. A quick PubMed search for "work life balance" brings up almost a thousand citations, with close to 400 having *surgeons* in the title, and half of these being specific to *female surgeons*. There are additional publications addressing specialties where women are least represented [4].

It is crucial to maintain the increasing awareness in the medical community of the need for work-life integration for female surgeons, as well as the negative effects on their performance if it is not achieved [5, 6]. Utilizing available resources helps female surgeons develop resilience and the ability to celebrate their personal and professional achievements with equal joy. Having professional accomplishments without being intentional about taking time to do self-care and engage in family life leads to an imbalance. Developing work-life integration requires intentional behavior to schedule time for personal wellness and development as carefully as surgeons schedule their clinic and OR days. This allows them to achieve success in their professional lives and also have personal fulfillment.

Conclusion

The integration of the personal and professional aspects of a surgeon's life should be approached with graciousness and a recognition of the need to adapt to circumstances. A deliberate approach to your own interpretation of work life integration is necessary to minimize the pressure placed on female surgeons by society. There is no one right way, though it is crucial to constantly be aware that your happiness and well-being are of utmost importance. Finding wholeness is attainable. Burnout should be prevented by having a fulfilling professional life while allowing for time to pursue hobbies and activities important to your wellness, as well as precious time with your loved ones.

Available Resources

1. Association of Women Surgeons website
2. American College of Surgeons: Surgeon Wellness - American Board of Surgery
3. Free apps as supported by your home institution (e.g., Calm, Headspace)
4. Mindful practice:

    https://www.mayoclinic.org/healthy-lifestyle/consumer-health/in-depth/mindfulness-exercises/art-200 46356

5. Free services and activities:

    Meditation
    Outside walks
    Library books

References

1. Hillert A, Albrecht A, Voderholzer U, 2020. The Burnout Phenomenon: A Résumé After More Than 15,000 Scientific Publications. Front Psychiatry 9;11:519237
2. Burn-out an "occupational phenomenon": International Classification of Diseases. WHO Burnout 2019:
3. Job burnout: How to spot it and take action—Mayo Clinic. Mayo Clinic, Job burnout: How to spot it and take action. 2023

4. Antonoff, M, Brown, L. Work-Life balance: the female cardiothoracic surgeon perspective. J Thorac Cardiovasc Surg 2015;150:1416-21

5. Yaghmour NA, Bynum WE IV, Hafferty FW, et al. Causes of death among US medical residents. JAMA Netw Open. 2025;8(5):e259238.

6. Moneme C, Obidike P, Yost J, Friel, C. How i do it: suicidal ideation during surgical training: is an innovative surgical trainee check ins program a part of the solution? J Surg Educ. 2023;80(10):1355-1357.

7. Brown C, Joseph B., Davis, K. Jurkovich, G., 2021. Modifiable factors to improve work-life balance for trauma surgeons. Journal of Acute care Surgery 90(1): p 122-128

8. Mindfulness exercises—Mayo Clinic

Chapter 11
Leadership Opportunities and Career Advancement

Stephanie Bonne

Introduction: Why Leadership?

In 2025, "Leadership" is a popular buzzword, and a goal that many surgeons of all genders and backgrounds strive for. Leadership, however, is a blanket term that can mean many things. We lead in the operating room, we lead in our institutions, as committee members and thought leaders, and we may even lead in our surgical organizations, medical schools, or health care systems. It's worthwhile, then, to unpack the reasons we want to be leaders and how that vision can drive our development.

Let's start with what leadership is not: it's not making the call schedule, or having a group of people who report to you who you command to bend to your will. It's not "bossing" people around or giving directives. It's also not "having a title" for the purposes of the title, rather than doing the work required of the role. If deep in your heart, this is why you want to lead, leadership will be difficult for you and difficult for the people around you, and you should take another look at whether leadership is the best way for you to contribute.

The best leaders begin with servant leadership and lead by example. This may mean taking an emergency call on a holiday so your partners can be with their families, or always being available as an extra layer of backup, or for a partner to call to talk through a challenging case. It also means that you need to exhibit the level of professionalism that you want your team to exhibit on your behalf, be as dedicated and available as you want them to be, and demonstrate the behaviors you want them to emulate. People, particularly junior to you or trainees, will be looking to your

S. Bonne (✉)
Professor of Surgery, Wake Forest University School of Medicine, Winston-Salem, NC, USA

Department of Surgery, Advocate Christ Medical Center, Oak Lawn, IL, USA
e-mail: Stephanie.bonne@aah.org

K. Yoon-Flannery et al. (eds.), *Women in Surgery*,
https://doi.org/10.1007/978-3-032-10971-2_11

example and be listening for the way you speak about others, be it doctors from other specialties, other leaders, or our multidisciplinary colleagues.

Good leaders draw on their experience and expertise to lay out a vision for what they want to build in the spaces that they lead, and then create space for others to execute that vision. When you are brought into a leadership role, the people who tasked you with this role rely on your expertise to craft a vision. Let's take being a division chief, for example, since that's probably the most visible leader to most academic surgeons. Surgical chairs invite division chiefs to lead their division because those chiefs understand the modern landscape of their particular subspecialty, but also either know or learn the local influences at the institution. This allows them to tailor the vision for the division to fit the priorities of the institutional leaders, while also helping those leaders understand modern practice, regulatory needs, and trends in patient care, education, and research.

Surgeons are particularly well-suited to lead health care efforts for several reasons. As individuals who practice broad specialties, surgeons have significant experience interacting with numerous areas of the hospital. Surgeons are found in the emergency department, interacting frequently with diagnostic testing departments, such as radiology and the laboratory, and in the intensive care units, inpatient units, and outpatient clinics. Additionally, surgeons are raised in a culture of leading the spaces they interact in. We are leaders in trauma resuscitation, in the operating room, and on our teams.

Becoming a Leader

When I was an early-career surgeon, I remember listening to a talk given by a prominent woman surgeon, who outlined her pathway into a position of significant influence in her organization, where she was an upper-level executive. She recalled seemingly serendipitous encounters in which she met key sponsors and mentors, who helped elevate her profile in the surgical world. I found this incredibly frustrating to listen to at the time. It seemed that she was recounting a fairy tale of chance encounters that put her in the right place at the right time to be tapped for ever-advancing roles, and I wondered if I even had a chance.

Over time, however, I learned that serendipity favors the prepared. Many people don't end up on the pathway they set out on, and many very accomplished leaders in surgery will tell you they took a circuitous path and ended up somewhere different from what they expected, myself included. When you are prepared, opportunities do seem to come to you rather unexpectedly, and if you have the skill set and the judgement to choose correctly, unexpected opportunities can become career-advancing in ways that were not anticipated. Preparation can also mean professional networking, being open to new ideas or projects, and taking on opportunities and completing projects. If you volunteer for a project or a committee, it is extremely important to complete the tasks and deliverables you sign up for, and be present at meetings for the efforts you've committed yourself to. This presence is incredibly important to taking the next steps in your leadership journey and earning credibility among your peers.

With that in mind, one suggestion is not to set or prepare for goals that are too far in the future, as life and career may take you in a different direction. For example, investing in a business degree as a resident or fellow because you think you may want to be a hospital executive could end up being a waste of time if you have a great research mentor, develop a prolific research career, and spend your life's work running a basic science lab. Or, you may get to the corporate leadership level, but by the time you do, your degree is outdated or obsolete. With that in mind, one strategy is to focus on the next step or the next five years. Ask yourself what skill set you currently possess, how you could contribute more or in a different or better way, and what gap in skill set you need in order to fill it. You may find at some point that you need an advanced degree, but it may be that you need a professional development course, or simply some more time and experience to hone your current skill set. Then, when you've achieved and mastered the next position, once again look around at the possible next steps, always thinking about how you can offer more to the next job, not just how you can get the next title.

The best time to advance to leadership is when you've accomplished much of what you want for yourself and are ready to support the growth and development of others. You should be at a point in your career where you don't need to apply for every grant, get every award, sit on every committee, or be at the podium at every meeting. When watching the people you lead accomplish these things is enough for your self-actualization, you are ready.

In the past several years, it has become more popular to pursue leadership training. Many surgical subspecialty organizations, medical organizations, and institutions offer leadership training courses that formalize the development of leadership skills. It has clearly become more of a mandate than previously to participate in training and be prepared to lead. Finding the right leadership course for your career path and timing leadership courses correctly is important, and therefore, it's important to pay careful attention to the scope and audience for the leadership class you plan to take. For example, academic-focused leadership courses may focus more on grants or leading education programs. Early career programs may focus on how to set goals, interact with others, and create agendas and reports. Executive leadership courses may focus more on finances, conflict management, or program development. Society leadership programs may be specifically dedicated to developing individuals to lead committees or efforts in that particular society and accomplish their mission.

Finally, when considering a formal leadership position in your institution, another institution, or in your specialty, it is imperative to understand how your success will be measured and what the tools are that you need to be successful. The tools and resources you need, when possible, should be negotiated up front, and there should be clear metrics and expectations for your success in your new role. For example, when taking on a service line medical directorship, you will want to ensure you have access to the data and metrics necessary to effect change and maintain quality, you will need data analysts or support staff who can help you enact change, and you will need the agency and authority to make necessary changes or decisions. Having responsibility without authority or decision-making capacity is a setup for failure. Having a leadership position without the time, compensation, or support staff needed to function in your role is also a setup for disaster.

Finally, not having a clearly defined set of metrics on which your success will be measured, and having these in writing, is another pathway to potential conflict or failure. One tool that is useful is SMART tools—your goals for your role should be specific, measurable, achievable, relevant, and time-bound. Good examples are "I will develop a quality improvement committee that meets 4 times per year and reviews at least 25 cases. This committee will also review 50% of existing clinical practice guidelines and create a practitioner dashboard for guideline adherence within 2 years." A poor example would be "I'm going to improve department quality."

Being a Good Leader in Your Position

Once you are in a leadership position, it is important to be thoughtful and deliberate with your role and your future development. Setting clear expectations for the performance of your team, while also developing trust and collegiality, can be a very difficult line to walk, particularly for women who are often subject to increased scrutiny of their "attitude and tone." It is very helpful to seek mentorship from those who understand your institutional culture as well as from those outside your field who may have more objective advice to help you manage your new role and oversee your team.

When in a leadership role, soliciting feedback regularly from key stakeholders is absolutely essential. This can be done informally, formally, or through evaluations such as a 360-evaluation, in which formal evaluations are distributed to those who work with you, as your leaders, as your direct reports, and as your peers. Whatever way you solicit feedback, it's important to remain objective, take feedback seriously and unemotionally, and try to understand how you can improve. Positive feedback should be regarded as behaviors that people want to see you continue. Negative feedback should be taken back to your mentors and discussed, with clear, SMART ways that you can work toward improvement.

Many leaders have found it advantageous to also have professional coaching. Rather than a mentor, who you seek to emulate, a coach can help you identify opportunities for improvement and develop improvement plans. Consider an athletic coach who identifies a weak left arm affecting an athlete's overall performance. That coach may recommend a weight-lifting and stretching program for that arm. Similarly, if a coach identifies that you have a gap—perhaps you are chronically late to meetings—they may help you identify strategies to improve, such as setting alarms, asking your assistant not to schedule meetings back to back, or building in breaks to your day for meals or unstructured time.

There are a number of practical strategies that a coach can help you identify, but there are some tips that are generally regarded as good practice for leaders. Here are some:

- Don't overschedule meetings. Not every issue needs a meeting; many can be handled by email, so use email and other communication when possible.
- When meetings are necessary, have an agenda. When possible, send out the agenda in advance so all your team members have an opportunity to prepare for the meeting and bring their contributions. Set an expectation that agendas are reviewed in advance and that individuals are prepared. If you are invited to a meeting without an agenda, ask for an agenda, citing that you prefer to come to meetings prepared to speak about the relevant issues. If you are unprepared or an agenda wasn't given, don't make decisions on the fly. You can always say that you would like time to research, consider, and discuss a course of action and regroup at a later date.
- Meet in person. Don't put anything in an email or say anything on a recorded Zoom line that you wouldn't want splashed across the front page of the New York Times. Everything is traceable; emails get inadvertently forwarded. Choose your words carefully and always maintain professionalism in your communications.
- Document your conversations when appropriate. For sensitive issues, like those related to personnel, or difficult conversations, send yourself an email summarizing a meeting when it's fresh in your mind, so you can revisit it later if needed. Emailing yourself is a great strategy when you want to refer to something later. It's also time-stamped.
- When important decisions are made, send a follow-up communication. It can be very appropriate to email an institutional leader after a meeting and say "thank you for meeting today and being committed to the advancement of our program. To recap—we discussed the need for this resource for our patients, and you committed to provide xxx by yyy date, so that we can move this initiative forward. We will be following our patient satisfaction scores in the next 2 quarters to review the anticipated success of this new program." Once again, time-stamping your information and outlining the expectations will provide clarity and accountability for all who are involved.
- Be deliberate and conscientious about your schedule. As mentioned above, by the time you are ready for leadership, you shouldn't feel the need to say yes to every opportunity that you are presented with. Review opportunities, decide if they will benefit you, and carefully craft your commitments to reflect your priorities, values, and what you love to do. When asked to be part of a committee or do a task, first ask yourself if it's required. If the answer is yes, then you have to do it. These are things that are contractual parts of your job, or things like medical records, expected committee obligations, etc. If something is optional, ask if it's helping you get where you want to be in 5 years. If the answer is yes, then do it. If the answer is no, try to delegate to someone else or politely decline. When declining, try to identify a surrogate or make a recommendation for another individual who may be interested.

- Schedule unstructured time, in particular if you work in an organization where others have access to your calendar. Block out time for things that are important, like family events, exercise, or hobbies. Schedule "desk time" and make sure your assistant knows that it's not to be infringed upon, so you have time to answer emails, catch up on paperwork, or simply have a cup of coffee and journal.
- Consider the importance of team building events, retreats, or facilitated strategic planning exercises. Most organizations have access to or have internal organizational psychology groups to support teams in the system. Having a regular opportunity to discuss team goals and values, developing a mission statement or a set of core values, and writing these down and displaying them in your team space can help ground the team and remind everyone that we all have the same goals in mind. This can also help alleviate disconnect between team members and also help direct resources toward the initiatives that are most important to your team. The strategic goals can vary widely. Some teams may be most committed to training the next generation of surgeons, while other teams may be more committed to basic science research. Other teams may have a top priority of providing as much care as possible to an underserved population. All of these are laudable goals, but making sure everyone is aligned with the overall team goals will help individuals understand how they can best contribute.

In summary, leadership can be both challenging and rewarding. Leadership offers us an opportunity to advocate for our profession and our patients in spaces where important decisions are being made, and therefore, surgeons should absolutely pursue leadership opportunities. There are structured opportunities to help you prepare for leadership and maintain your skills, and seeking constant mentorship and feedback can help you be successful and have a meaningful and lasting impact on your team and institution.

Chapter 12
Military Surgery

Kristen Knapp

In the fall of 2019, I was a fourth-year medical student buried deep in an existential crisis about what to do with my life. I was torn not only between specialties—should I pursue surgery, my true passion, or emergency medicine, which boasted an easier lifestyle and shorter training—but also paths in clinical medicine; was it finally time to join the military, or would I be signing my life away?

I'd always planned to join the military at some point, having grown up with mentors, family, and friends in all branches of the armed forces. There are many points in a medical career at which a physician can join the military, and I had considered all of them. For those ready to fully immerse in military medicine, there's the highly selective Uniformed Services University of the Health Sciences (USUHS)—the military's medical school. Acceptance into USUHS, which is highly competitive, incurs a 7-year active duty service obligation in the Army, Navy, Air Force, or U.S. Public Health Service after completion of residency. Of note, the Marines do not have a medical force but instead are served by Navy medicine. Students enjoy the benefits of active duty pay, housing allowance, tuition-free medical education, and early exposure and immersion in military life. Unfortunately, with my unconventional academic background and no prior military service, I was not offered an interview.

Thankfully, there are other ways to join the military medical force as a medical student. The Health Professions Scholarship Program (HPSP) is available to any student accepted to a US civilian medical school, through all branches of the military—Army, Navy, and Air Force—as well as the U.S. Public Health Service. When I was accepted to medical school at the University of Virginia, I engaged with recruiters from every branch. The benefits of the HPSP program are the same

K. Knapp (✉)
Department of Surgery, Cooper University Hospital, Cooper Medical School of Rowan University, Camden, NJ, USA
e-mail: knapp-kristen@cooperhealth.edu

K. Yoon-Flannery et al. (eds.), *Women in Surgery*,
https://doi.org/10.1007/978-3-032-10971-2_12

regardless of the service chosen—scholarship recipients are commissioned as second lieutenants in their branch of choice, which pays all medical tuition and fees, and receive a monthly stipend of over $2500. Depending on the branch, students may also receive a signing bonus and 45 days of active duty pay. In return, for each year the scholarship is accepted, students incur a year of active duty commitment. During medical school, students are required to spend 45 days a year in active duty. Between years 1 and 2, the required basic officer training fulfills this requirement. For the remaining clinical years, rotations at military hospitals count towards active duty time, and students are paid as such.

Upon graduating from medical school, students may apply to both military and civilian residency programs in most cases. However, their specialty and residency choice can be affected by the needs of the military. In specialties where military need is high (internal medicine, pediatrics, emergency medicine, ob-gyn, and general surgery), it would be extremely unlikely to be denied entry into the specialty of your choice. However, should one desire a less common specialty, such as ENT or ophthalmology, if the military currently had a surplus of physicians in this subspecialty and low predicted future need for this specialty, the student could be pushed into another specialty for which the military had a high need. Similarly, if a student desired to match into a civilian residency, but military residency spots remained unfilled, that student might be denied the opportunity to join the civilian match. In this unusual situation, the student would have the option to either enter a specialty or residency according to their branch's needs or accept a GMO position (graduate medical officer) for a year or more, then re-attempt the match in the future. A GMO provides primary care in their branch of choice and an opportunity to support soldiers, sailors, marines, or airmen in operational units.

By the beginning of medical school, I had been accepted for HPSP in the Army, Navy, and Air Force. Having no idea what specialty I might find myself attracted to, however, I did not accept my commission for fear of having my specialty choice reassigned or needing to complete multiple GMO tours without a promise of eventual acceptance into my residency of choice. That being said, all my friends from medical school in the Army, Navy, and Air Force HPSP spoke highly of their experiences and are now in specialties and residency programs they love. By the time residency application rolled around in my fourth year of medical school, I was beginning to feel like maybe I had "missed the boat" as I watched my HPSP classmates navigating military rotations, joining in on enriching field exercises, and reaping all the other benefits HPSP has to offer.

Thankfully, during this time, I learned there are yet more ways to join the military as a resident. All branches of the military have a reserve incentive program available to residents in eligible specialties: the Army STRAP (Specialized TRaining Assistance Program), Navy TMS (Training in Medical Specialties), and Air Force Reserve Stipend Program all offer a direct route into the military as a reserve officer. All boast a stipend of ~$2500 a month during residency, and most offer loan repayment up to $250,000. Time spent in residency contributes to retirement. In return, the resident accrues 2 years of reserve service commitment for every 1 year the stipend is accepted. Upon graduation or residency, they will enter the civilian work-force, but must remain ready to deploy as a reserve physician.

Around the time I began to consider the Army's STRAP program, I was rotating as an M4 in the Cooper University Hospital Emergency Department in Camden, NJ. I found myself torn between applying emergency medicine, with its comfortable lifestyle and short training time, or surgery—a daunting commitment, but the specialty I had found most fulfilling by far. I chose to rotate at Cooper in an effort to convince myself that emergency medicine was the field for me. However, I found myself distracted—drawn to the trauma bay and ORs—and disinterested by the medical problems I encountered in the ED. I wanted to fix things that were broken, not just temporize. As such, I found myself reading the CV of LTC John Chovanes on the Cooper Department of Surgery website. Dr. Chovanes' background stood out to me as similar to mine, and his career path had taken him to many of the destinations I was considering. Prior to medical school, Dr. Chovanes had been an EMT, flight paramedic, and nurse. He went on to complete both medical school and surgical residency at the Philadelphia College of Osteopathic Medicine and the Trauma and Critical Care Fellowship at the University of Pennsylvania. Just as I was considering, he had joined the Army Reserves as a surgical resident, almost 20 years earlier. Needless to say, I immediately reached out—desperate for advice from someone who had walked a similar path.

If you've spent any time in the medical profession, you know that getting a response to a cold email by an attending surgeon is nothing short of a miracle. But he did, and several days later, I found myself sitting in the "Embassy," the hub for Military, Diplomatic, and Field Surgical Affairs at Cooper Hospital. I was expecting to meet a jaded and bitter doctor who would tell me, like many others had, to steer clear of the profession. Instead, I was met by an energetic surgeon, passionate about his work both at home and abroad. He regaled me with stories from residency and fellowship and told me about his many rewarding tours of duty since joining the reserves in 2001: trauma surgeon with the 325th Combat Support Hospital on Contingency Operating Base Speicher in Tikrit, Iraq, 2007; trauma surgeon and the Deputy Commander of Clinical Services at Forward Operating Base Salerno in Khowst, Afghanistan, 2010 and 2012; and trauma surgeon at Camp Manion with the 948th Forward Surgical Team during the Third Battle of Fallujah, 2016. He shared many of the interesting clinical challenges he encountered, such as removing an unexploded rocket-propelled grenade from a U.S. Soldier, for which he received the Army Commendation Medal for Meritorious Service.

Furthermore, he explained that rather than hurting his civilian career, his position in the Army had allowed him to build Cooper Hospitals "Military, Diplomatic, and Field Surgical Affairs" department, for which he is the Chief Military Surgeon. The department hosts the Military Civilian Trauma Team Training Program, an embedded group of military physicians, nurses, paramedics, and APPs, who work and train together at Cooper to be best prepared for deployment, and also trains hundreds of Special Operations Combat Medics (SOCM's) from the U.S. Army Special Forces and Rangers, Navy SEALS, and Marine Recon, army medics, U.S. State Department medical personal, and more. He also told me about the unique opportunity to work alongside other surgical specialties, such as ENT and ob-gyn physicians. In all his stories, this appealed to me the most—the opportunity to work together with a diverse team, in an austere environment, committed to a common goal.

Needless to say, I left our meeting with the reassurance I needed to charge forward. I matched in general surgery at Cooper Hospital and was commissioned as a Captain in the Army Reserves soon after. Now, almost 4 years later, I've yet to regret the decision. On the practical side of things, having some extra income during residency has allowed me to provide my family with a much better quality of life during training. More significantly, being in the army has opened up a world of opportunities during training, such as attending military conferences and courses, training medics and police, publishing in military publications, and more, and has never interfered with my residency duties. I've met incredible teachers, such as Colonel Kirby Gross, who joined the team at Cooper just as my residency began and recently retired from the army at age 70 after over 20 years of service and ten deployments. I also had the opportunity to start our medical school's Military Medical Interest Group, and the experience of mentoring young military physicians just embarking on their careers has been deeply rewarding. This year, I promoted the first group of students who joined MMIG as M1s at their Graduation Ceremony, and I was especially honored to promote Captain Sheth (Air Force), who is now my intern in the Cooper General Surgery Residency.

Thousands of years ago, the father of medicine Hippocrates stated "He who wishes to be a surgeon should go to war." So many of our medical advances have stemmed from conflict, and the innovation spurred from the human damage war incurs. Being in the military will put me at the forefront of this wave of innovation. Most importantly, however, knowing that I will have a long military commitment ahead of me provides even more motivation to get the most out of my training. Knowing that I'll be responsible for leading a team charged with protecting the lives of our injured soldiers, sailors, marines, and airmen, as well as injured host nationals and even opposition forces, in resource-poor scenarios, often far from additional help and expertise, drives me to soak up every opportunity to advance my knowledge. Our young men and women who put themselves in harm's way to defend our nation deserve the absolute best care medicine has to offer, from the most dedicated team. If this sentiment strikes a cord in your heart as well, consider joining us.

Part IV
Building a Practice

Chapter 13
Your Partners Could Be Your Lifeline

Margo Carlin and Asanthi Ratnasekera

Choosing the right practice and partners is a fundamental aspect of professional growth for any surgeon and carries particular significance for female surgeons due to the unique challenges we often face within the medical field. Systemic biases, a lack of representation among leadership, and the need to balance demanding work schedules with personal and family commitments are silent challenges that can insidiously decrease professional enjoyment and lead to burnout. Finding a supportive practice environment is essential to nurture your talent, foster professional relationships, and ensure your long-term success because who you work with is equally as important as where you work. Here, we will explore some key elements you should consider when exploring new job opportunities, with an emphasis on interview techniques and red flags to watch for that may indicate a dysfunctional environment.

Factors such as work culture, mentorship opportunities, career development pathways, and personal support systems can greatly impact a woman's career trajectory in surgery [1]. A positive work culture promotes respect, collaboration, and diversity and enhances job satisfaction, retention, and overall professional development. Mentorship opportunities are crucial, as mentors provide guidance, encouragement, and sponsorship that female surgeons need to navigate clinical challenges and career advancement [2]. Without effective mentorship, many women may find it difficult to access leadership roles or earn recognition for their contributions.

M. Carlin (✉)
Department of Surgery, Christiana Care, Newark, DE, USA
e-mail: margo.carlin@christianacare.org

A. Ratnasekera
Associate Trauma Medical Director, Assistant Professor of Surgery, Christiana Care, Newark, DE, USA
e-mail: margo.carlin@christianacare.org

K. Yoon-Flannery et al. (eds.), *Women in Surgery*,
https://doi.org/10.1007/978-3-032-10971-2_13

Career development is another pivotal concern; practices that actively support continuing education, training, and advancement opportunities can empower you to reach your full potential. Moreover, personal support systems—including colleagues who understand and accommodate the complexities of work-life balance—can make a significant difference in a surgeon's ability to thrive both personally and professionally. Although some women may not need work-life balance to feel personally and professionally satisfied, it is ok to prioritize this aspect of your life if this is important to you [3].

Effective questioning during an interview can reveal deeper insights into the work environment and dynamics of the workplace to provide a clearer picture of the practice's culture. These interview techniques can help you gauge the compatibility of a practice before you commit to a long-term contract. Reflect on your own values and career aspirations before you interview or meet with potential partners. Considering what is most important to you will help you find a good fit without compromising your needs. Is work-life balance important? (i.e., Do you wish for flexible hours or part-time work? Or are you fully committed to a busy surgical career?) What kind of professional development factors do you wish to pursue (i.e., availability of continuing education on and off campus, reimbursement for scientific activities like conferences, mentorship opportunities)?

Every practice has its own unique and established culture, and you will not thrive in every workplace. Workplace culture is generally set long before your interview, and your time with the practice is unlikely to change an established mindset. It may not be possible to assess a group's priorities on things like inclusivity, support, and respect for all patients and staff members from a single interview, so do not blame or self-depreciate if it is revealed over time that your values contrast or you misjudged a work environment [4, 5]. Your needs and principles are important and are a priority, and if they are not honored in your workplace, it will affect your personal and professional life [6]. Every practice culture is distinct in that workplace, and practice patterns vary across different groups and regions. Different practices are not inferior practices. The way science advances is by alternative thought, so bringing your unique perspective and training can help a practice thrive. If your partners do not respect your training, ideas, or patient approach, that particular practice is not the right fit for you.

Furthermore, targeted questions not only help reveal the dynamics of the practice but also give insight into the overall attitude toward collaboration and growth. Opportunities for mentorship are essential for career advancement at every stage of your career, regardless of whether you are a junior, mid-career, or senior attending, and asking interviewers to describe mentorship opportunities or relationships within the practice can help with transparency of career development. To help find your fit, ask interviewers to characterize existing measures in place to ensure inclusivity and support among colleagues. How are decisions made within the practice? Is input from all partners valued, or is there a hierarchical approach? Female surgeons with family obligations often face challenges balancing schedules, so do not hesitate to ask what kind of policies are in place to support partners who have personal commitments outside of work. Your quality of life is important, and although you may find it reasonable to compromise mentorship and work culture for a schedule that fits your lifestyle, a toxic workplace will eventually affect you at home. It is important to ask questions to help you assess whether the environment is supportive and collaborative or if it might be structured in a way that could inhibit your growth and happiness [7].

Paying attention to how things are said during interviews is just as important as what is said. The behavior and mannerisms of the partners can often reveal much about a practice's culture. Taking note of how existing partners interact with each other can provide insight into the collegiality of the group. Do they show respect and support, or do they appear competitive with or dismissive of each other? Be particularly alert to negative comments or "jokes" about current or previous partners or other employees within the group. This can help shine light on a toxic and/or blame culture, which is not only physically and emotionally exhausting, but can ultimately hurt you professionally if your partners denigrate you in a shared network or predispose you to litigation if partners document their opinions in official medical records.

Additionally, although it is not possible to identify every red flag from a single interview, it is important to pay attention to the ones that you do see, as these concerns can blossom into the detriment of your career once you are well into your contract. For example, a high turnover rate is a red flag that typically indicates a toxic work environment. Turnover can be easy to identify through frequent and recurrent recruitment ads on job boards or by asking how long people usually stay in their position with the group. If you receive an answer such as "the length of the contract," this usually means a high turnover rate. Conduct informal research about the group and the hospital by speaking to previous employees or trainees through your network. Furthermore, a lack of female representation among the partners or in hospital leadership roles can signify systemic issues regarding support and advancement for female surgeons [8]. By recognizing these signs early, you can try to avoid practices that may impede your professional growth or contribute to dissatisfaction and burnout.

Once you secure a position you love, intermittently assessing long-term compatibility is crucial, especially since the dynamics of a surgical practice can change over time. Ensure that your professional goals align with the vision and growth of the practice. Make sure there are ongoing opportunities within the practice to help you grow professionally through mentorship programs, research activities, or the education of medical students, residents, or fellows. A partnership that thrives on the collective success of the group and celebrates the achievements of each individual not only promotes innovation and morale but also guarantees personal and professional contentment.

The right partnership will not only enhance your skills and advance your career but also foster a supportive and satisfying work environment. Identifying suitable partners in a surgical practice is a multifaceted process, especially for female surgeons navigating a historically male-dominated field. It involves a comprehensive understanding of personal and professional objectives, a proactive approach during the interview process, and a keen awareness of the subtleties in workplace interactions and attitudes. By understanding your values, asking insightful questions during interviews, observing interpersonal dynamics, recognizing red flags, networking wisely, and assessing long-term compatibility, you can make informed decisions to mitigate burnout and enhance the longevity of your surgical vocation. By employing these strategies, female surgeons can significantly enhance their chances of finding a supportive, progressive, and growth-oriented practice, ultimately fostering a successful and fulfilling career in surgery.

References

1. Turfah, M., & Kwakye, G. (2023). Negotiation and Career Advancement: How Can We Continue to Advance Women in Academic Surgery, What Are the Barriers They Are Facing, and What Can We Do to Overcome Them? *Clinics in colon and rectal surgery*, *36*(5), 321–326. https://doi.org/10.1055/s-0043-1763520
2. Mahendran, G. N., Walker, E. R., Bennett, M., & Chen, A. Y. (2022). Qualitative Study of Mentorship for Women and Minorities in Surgery. *Journal of the American College of Surgeons*, *234*(3), 253–261. https://doi.org/10.1097/XCS.0000000000000059
3. Brown, C. V. R., Joseph, B. A., Davis, K., & Jurkovich, G. J. (2021) Modifiable factors to improve work-life balance for trauma surgeons. *The journal of trauma and acute care surgery*, *90*(1), 122–128. https://doi.org/10.1097/TA.0000000000002910
4. Pei, K. Y., & Cochran, A. (2019). Workplace Bullying Among Surgeons-the Perfect Crime. *Annals of surgery*, *269*(1), 43–44. https://doi.org/10.1097/SLA.0000000000003018
5. Contreras, N., Essig, R., Magarinos, J., & Pereira, S. (2024). Abuse, Bullying, Harassment, Discrimination, and Allyship in Cardiothoracic Surgery. *Thoracic surgery clinics*, *34*(3), 239–247. https://doi.org/10.1016/j.thorsurg.2024.04.001
6. Lund, S., D'Angelo, J. D., Jogerst, K., Warner, S. G., Busch, R., & D'Angelo, A. D. (2022). Revealing hidden experiences: Gendered microaggressions and surgical faculty burnout. *Surgery*, *172*(3), 885–889. https://doi.org/10.1016/j.surg.2022.04.032
7. Schizas, D., Papapanou, M., Routsi, E., Mastoraki, A., Lidoriki, I., Zavras, N., Avgerinos, D. V., Lazaris, A. M., & Tsaroucha, A. (2022). Career barriers for women in surgery. *The surgeon : journal of the Royal Colleges of Surgeons of Edinburgh and Ireland*, *20*(5), 275–283. https://doi.org/10.1016/j.surge.2021.11.008
8. Stephens, E. H., Heisler, C. A., Temkin, S. M., & Miller, P. (2020). The Current Status of Women in Surgery: How to Affect the Future. *JAMA surgery*, *155*(9), 876–885. https://doi.org/10.1001/jamasurg.2020.0312

Chapter 14
Marketing and Branding

Beth B. DuPree

Introduction

As a general surgeon, now identifying as a breast surgeon, with over 35 years' experience, I have lived through the evolution of branding and marketing in healthcare. When I began practicing as a general surgeon, patients did not have access to to online resources such as search engines, websites or social media platforms including Instagram, X, LinkedIn or "Dr. Google". The only marketing you received was when you made the news cycle, whether good, bad, or indifferent. Without seeking notoriety, I made the front page of my local paper 6 months into my surgery career in an article on working professional moms. The hospital's communication department had set up the interview, and I didn't think anything of it, so I mentioned it to my partners, and it was no big deal. No big deal until the Sunday paper came out a few months later and the half-page color picture of me brushing my 2-year-old's teeth in his Mickey Mouse ears hit the newsstand. My senior partner in the group was elated as he viewed it as free advertising for our surgical practice. "Any press is money in the bank for the practice, positive press is priceless." The younger male associate expressed concern, noting that he did not perceive my role as a surgeon-mother to be materially different than his and felt the article was unnecessary. It was at that moment that I became keenly aware of how an individual's "branding"/ marketing can impact a group and ultimately a health system's image and reputation.

B. B. DuPree (✉)
Redeemer Health, Southampton, PA, USA
e-mail: bbdmouth@gmail.com

K. Yoon-Flannery et al. (eds.), *Women in Surgery*,
https://doi.org/10.1007/978-3-032-10971-2_14

Social Media Policies and Institutional Considerations

Before you begin to brand or market anything about yourself or your practice, you need to carefully review and adhere to your health system and your employer's set of policies and procedures regarding the use of social media. Within professional environments, seeking organizational approval prior to posting is far safer than relying on forgiveness after the fact. Having used both approaches in my life, I would suggest obtaining permission unless you are prepared to potentially lose your job for not following the rules and regulations set out by your employers communications department. In the United States of America, we do have *the First Amendment* right to freedom of speech but that right is a personal right. As an employed physician, your online words and actions may affect your employment, credentialing and professional reputation.

- Understand your employer's social media policies and procedures
- Define the audience you want to reach
- Identify what differentiates you from other surgeons

Brand Development

The next step is to determine or create your "brand." Begin by developing a list of your talents, strengths, and values that you hope to share with the world. My brand initially emerged organically rather than through deliberate planning. From the outset, I had no interest in social media, particularly Facebook, until my health system nominated me for Philadelphia Magazine's Philly Health Hero in 2010. The nomination and voting for the award happened on Facebook, so I ultimately conceded to the communications department and created a Facebook account. They saw this visibility as "free advertising" for the health system. It took me a few years to actually make conscious decisions about branding. I hired a graphic designer to create my brand logo.

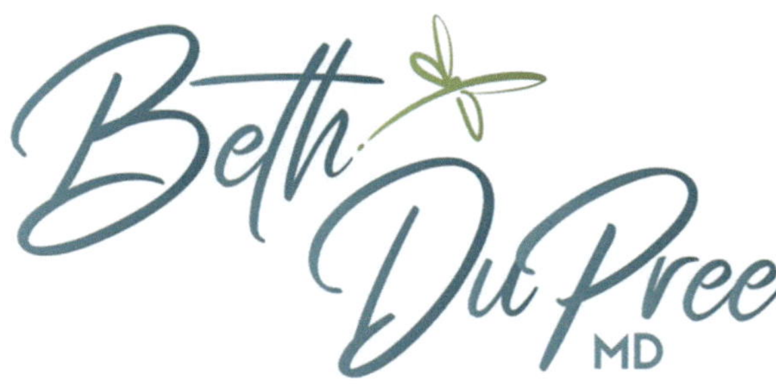

Your logo should reflect your personality, and you need to love it! If you really want to "brand" yourself, you need to be consistent across all of your social media accounts, email signatures, collateral materials, and your website. When you create or update your accounts, use your logo, an up-to-date headshot, and a background photo that connects all of your accounts. When you create your tagline, add a disclaimer that your posts are your own opinions and not medical advice. Adhere to the policies and procedures of your organization. Grow your followers organically with content.

Marketing Recommendations

Content suggestions

- Connect posts with your practice or organization using appropriate tags
- Develop engaging content supported by a curated list of topics
- Short videos enhance engagement (orient phone landscape or portrait based upon where you are posting)
- Maintain structured posting schedules, content management platforms are helpful
- Enhance your skills through courses from marketing experts live or on demand

Marketing Guru Todd Hartley was my online mentor and I highly recommend his course

- Master AI content creationbecome the rockstar of your niche
- Todd Hartley Social Super Star

- Rehearse then record professional quality videos and review them before posting to ensure clarity and confidence
- Use conscise, well-crafted quotations that reinforce your message
- Highlight your accomplishments
- Include a call to action (publicize podcasts, talks, and your upcoming events).

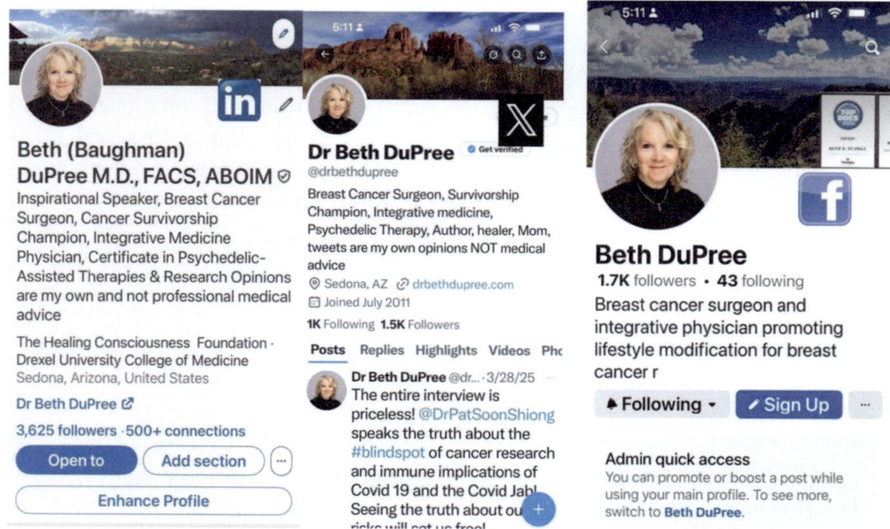

Conclusion

You have agency and autonomy of your beliefs and practices, but they may differ from those of your health system. By adhering to your institutional polices, identifying their core values, and planning online engagement deliberately, you can build a strong, authentic professional and trusted brand. Thoughtful planning and communication is essential particularly in digital spaces. If you fail to plan, then plan to fail. Think, rethink, and review before you post! Be a conscious responder, not a reactor. Simply liking a post, commenting on a post, let alone sharing a post can get you labeled, cancelled, and potentially fired. Actions have consequences, and we have witnessed physicians lose their jobs over COVID treatment controversies and the war in the Middle East.

DOCTOR SUES NYU AFTER BEING FIRED FOR SOCIAL MEDIA POSTS ON WAR IN MIDDLE EAST

NYU Langone Health | source: **ajay_suresh**

After a Palestinian doctor at New York University was fired for posting Instagram messages supporting Hamas, a Jewish physician at the school was fired for posts criticizing anti-Israel protesters. The second doctor has sued the university for wrongful termination and discrimination.

Patients, colleagues, and potential future employers can surf the internet and all of your social media engagement and learn a lot about who you are and what you believe. Unless you plan to quit your "day" job and become a paid influencer, you need to maintain control of your social media presence and at least approve all posts. Before you hit POST… remember, once shared, digital content becomes part of your permanent online record.

Chapter 15
Knowing When It's Time to Leave

Mckenzie Rowe and Paula Ferrada

Introduction: Finding Your Fit and Facing Change

A career in surgery is as much about skill and perseverance as it is about finding the right environment to thrive. The journey is often marked by periods of immense growth but also by moments of reflection—times when you must evaluate whether your current workplace aligns with your personal and professional values. Knowing when to leave is not just about dissatisfaction; it is about recognizing when a place no longer serves your growth, well-being, or career aspirations.

One of my mentors told me about a time he found himself at a crossroads. Despite enjoying his work, he noticed he began to feel stifled by a lack of supportive leadership and a workplace whose values were misaligned with his own. Conversations with trusted mentors and allies helped him recognize that staying out of loyalty or fear of change would not serve his long-term goals. His story, like many others, highlights the importance of strategic decision-making in career transitions.

M. Rowe (✉)
Department of Surgery, Inova Fairfax Health, Falls Church, VA, USA
e-mail: Mckenzie.Rowe@inova.org

P. Ferrada
Department of Surgery Inova Fairfax Medical Campus, Falls Church, VA, USA

Medical Director Perioperative Services IFMC, Falls Church, VA, USA

Division and System Chief for Trauma and Acute Care Surgery Inova Healthcare System, Falls Church, VA, USA

University of Virginia School of Medicine, Charlottesville, VA, USA

ELAM class 2020, Falls Church, VA, USA
e-mail: Paula.Ferrada@inova.org

K. Yoon-Flannery et al. (eds.), *Women in Surgery*,
https://doi.org/10.1007/978-3-032-10971-2_15

This chapter delves into the critical decision-making process involved in leaving a workplace. It explores key indicators that suggest when it might be time to move on, strategies for protecting yourself in challenging environments, and how to transition effectively into a role that better aligns with your goals. By leveraging mentorship, recognizing workplace toxicity, and learning from adversity, you can ensure that each career move is a step toward professional fulfillment.

Finding Mentors and Allies

A strong network of mentors and allies is indispensable in navigating career transitions. These relationships provide guidance, support, insight, and opportunities that can shape your professional trajectory.

How to Identify and Cultivate Mentorship

Mentorship is more than just seeking advice from senior colleagues—it is about forming meaningful relationships with individuals *whose values align with yours*. A good mentor is someone who provides honest, constructive feedback, guides you in career progression, and helps you assess your potential within your current role. They also offer insight into industry trends and job opportunities.

Seeking mentors *beyond your immediate work environment*—through professional organizations, conferences, LinkedIn, and alumni networks—broadens your perspective and opens new doors. One of my best mentors and coaches is actually our Education Director, who is a social worker by training. Because we align in our values, I am able to talk through career decisions with her and get honest feedback on how it might go along with my overall professional and personal goals. Additionally, *maintaining connections* with past mentors ensures you have ongoing guidance throughout your career and can help to identify outside opportunities.

Allies in the Workplace: Why They Matter

Allies within your workplace serve as *immediate support systems*. While mentors provide long-term guidance, allies help navigate day-to-day challenges. They can be peers, supervisors, or individuals in different departments who share your values and advocate for your success.

Building strong alliances involves identifying colleagues who align with your professional values, engaging in reciprocal support, having an open dialogue about workplace opportunities, and joining or creating professional groups to foster collaboration. When faced with the decision to leave a place, their insights can help you weigh your options with clarity and confidence.

The Role of Mentors and Allies in Decision-Making

By cultivating mentors and allies, you develop a *support network* that empowers you to make informed career decisions. These relationships not only provide professional guidance but also emotional and strategic support when facing difficult career choices. If you find yourself in an unsupportive environment, your mentors and allies can be instrumental in helping you navigate challenges and determine if leaving is the best course of action.

Knowing When You Are Not Safe and How to Strategize

This extends beyond physical well-being. Psychological safety—the ability to express ideas, ask questions, and challenge the status quo without fear of retribution—is equally important [1]. Signs that you may be in an unsafe environment include (1) consistent *gaslighting* or manipulation, (2) fear of speaking up due to *retaliation*, (3) *hostile leadership*, or (4) a culture that fosters *discrimination* and harassment [2, 3].

One of my good friends is a surgical resident who experienced a toxic work environment. Despite having strong allies and mentors at this prior program, she was repeatedly overlooked for opportunities and was not supported in her career goals by her Program Director. She wasn't sure how best to leave her situation.

Strategies for Navigating an Unsafe Environment

If you consistently feel *mentally drained, undervalued, or threatened, it may be time to leave*. If you find yourself in a toxic workplace, take the following steps:

- *Document everything:* Keep records of interactions, emails, and incidents.
- *Secure support:* Identify trusted allies who can vouch for you.
- *Know your rights:* Familiarize yourself with workplace policies and legal protections.
- *Plan your exit:* A strategic departure minimizes disruption to your career.

Recognizing when an environment is harmful—and acting on that realization—is an essential skill for long-term career success.

How to Protect Yourself

Leaving a workplace, particularly under difficult circumstances, requires careful planning. Protecting yourself requires a proactive approach:

- *Keep your job search confidential* until you have secured a new position.
- *Build financial flexibility* to ease the transition. Build an emergency fund that allows for flexibility.
- *Exit gracefully* to avoid burning bridges even in difficult circumstances; reputation follows you.
- *Secure references early* to obtain recommendation letters while relationships are strong.

This friend discreetly networked and found a program that was a better fit. She made sure to leave her program on good terms and was able to transition into another program that supported her career aspirations. A well-planned exit ensures you leave on your terms, safeguarding your professional integrity while setting yourself up for success.

Learning from your "Enemies"

Difficult workplace experiences, including *challenging colleagues, difficult supervisors, or competitive environments*, offer invaluable lessons. Exposure to both effective and ineffective leadership can help shape your own approach and allow you to seek environments that will be better suited for you. Adversity also builds resilience, enhances emotional intelligence, and clarifies your values [4].

When I have endured difficult attendings, senior residents, or even just people above me in organizations, it has taught me a lot about how I DON'T want to lead and the personalities that I would not want to work with in the future. Now, when I am in leadership roles and as I progress in my career, I prioritize fostering an inclusive and supportive environment focused on growth. I view these experiences as stepping stones to create and find a better professional future that fits my needs and values.

Conclusion: Making the Right Decision

Deciding to leave a place is never easy, but *recognizing when to move on and doing so strategically* can make all the difference. By fostering strong networks, identifying unsafe environments, protecting yourself, and learning from difficult experiences, you can transition smoothly into a workplace that fosters your growth and well-being.

Your career journey should be about more than survival—it should be about thriving in a space where you are valued, challenged, and supported. With the right preparation and mindset, you can navigate career transitions confidently and find a place where you truly belong.

References

1. Edmondson, A. (1999). Psychological Safety and Learning Behavior in Work Teams. *Administrative Science Quarterly, 44*(2), 350-383.
2. Pedulla, D. (2020). Diversity and Inclusion Efforts That Really Work. *Harvard Business Review.* Retrieved from https://hbr.org/2020/05/diversity-and-inclusion-efforts-that-really-work
3. Schein, E. H. (2010). *Organizational Culture and Leadership.* Jossey-Bass.
4. Goleman, D. (2006). *Emotional Intelligence: Why It Can Matter More Than IQ.* Bantam Books.

Chapter 16
Breaking Barriers in Academic Surgery

Elinore J. Kaufman

Introduction

A life in academic surgery is replete with extraordinary privileges, not just the privilege to, usually, live comfortably with job security and ample pay, but also the privilege of intimacy with the human body and the privilege to be with patients at their worst moments and to help them heal. I expected these privileges and was already able to appreciate them during surgical training. But when I finally transitioned from trainee to attending, I encountered another advantage of this profession. Although there are numerous pressures and demands upon an academic surgeon, I found I also had quite a bit of freedom to shape my professional life to my liking. I was able to explore the balance of clinical, academic, educational, and administrative pursuits. This sudden onset of flexibility allowed me to renew my understanding of health, broadly defined, and how I might contribute to it from my position within surgery.

The clinical care we work to master accounts for only approximately 20% of individual health outcomes. And half of that is access to care, leaving us, the treating clinicians, with only 10% for which we can take credit [1]. While all conditions of health and disease reflect social and structural conditions, this is particularly obvious in my field of trauma surgery. Every injury we treat is, on at least some level, preventable, and therefore, every injury we treat was caused at least in part by the absence of preventive measures, be they safety features of a vehicle or road, protective policies, or life opportunities that could have prevented a violent encounter.

The privileges of academic surgery allow me to attempt to broaden my contribution—to make a dent in some of the other structural and social

E. J. Kaufman (✉)
Assistant Professor of Surgery, University of Pennsylvania, Philadelphia, PA, USA
e-mail: elinore.kaufman@pennmedicine.upenn.edu

K. Yoon-Flannery et al. (eds.), *Women in Surgery*,
https://doi.org/10.1007/978-3-032-10971-2_16

83

determinants of health that hit my patients so hard. The mission of advocacy has become part of my mission as a surgeon and of my academic career.

Surgeons as Advocates

To provide high-quality care, all surgeons must function on some level as advocates—for our patients to get the care they need, for our services to get the resources necessary to function, for our trainees to get access to educational resources, for ourselves to get OR time, and for our profession. But we also have the opportunity, and, maybe, the obligation, to take this further and become advocates for change— for a better society. As surgeons, we build relationships of trust and intimacy with our patients and their families. We take part in and bear witness to their stories from up close. The world might be a better place if people in positions of power did the same—if they heard directly from our patients. But patients don't always have the time, interest, bandwidth, or, unfortunately, social capital to reach the decision makers whose decisions influence their lives. As physicians, we can sometimes bridge that gap, carrying the stories we experience in healthcare to the halls of power, advocating for better quality of healthcare, better access to care, or a new way of providing care. We can also advocate for health-promoting resources that can improve well-being for individuals, families, and communities; for justice within and beyond the profession (Fig. 16.1).

Advocacy can take place in a single interaction, for example, pushing for a patient with food insecurity who is being discharged home to have access to healthy food; in an institution, to establish a foodbank for similar patients, like the one at Boston Medical Center [2, 3]. Advocating within a professional society can lead to

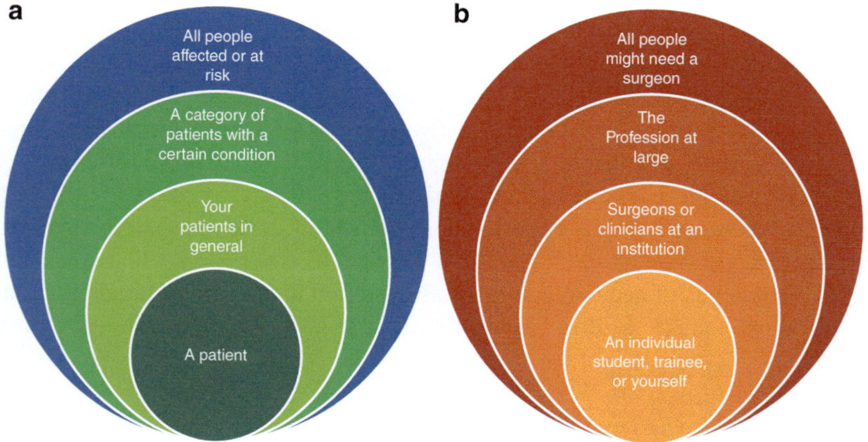

Fig. 16.1 Levels of advocacy motivated by experiences in healthcare. (**a**) Patient-focused, (**b**) Profession-focused

advocacy at a larger scale, if the society can support a particular position—such as equitable parental leave for surgical trainees [4]. Advocating at the community, local, state, and federal levels by working with community groups and policy makers can contribute to change at a larger scale.

Although I believe that advocacy can be an important part of an academic surgical career and that surgeons can be strong advocates, we are unlikely to develop comprehensive expertise in these strategies. The best advocacy is likely done in collaboration and in community, with the humility and patience to recognize that change is slow, but with the agility and persistence to respond to new opportunities or needs.

The Goal of Advocacy: Policy Change

Advocacy doesn't have to be political, but if it goes beyond the individual, it probably does involve policy. Policy can be federal, state, or local law, or the way these laws are implemented. But policy also exists at the level of the institution—a healthcare system, department, or professional society, and structures the answers to questions that affect issues we care about. If there is something you care about—the thing—policy can dictate whether that thing is allowed; whether it is incentivized, encouraged, or discouraged; whether it is required; and in what circumstances. Importantly, policy often dictates who pays for the thing, if the thing is a treatment or resource, and who has access to it. Policy also always contributes to the broader social and environmental context that contributes to or detracts from your thing of interest. And advocating for and against policies along these various axes can be an important way to make a difference.

Examples in Surgery

There are countless inspiring examples of surgeons working toward policy and social change at all scales. Some are directly related to patient care, such as the role that transplant surgeons take on in advocating for equitable organ allocation. Todd Wider was a plastic surgeon in Long Island, New York, who performed a breast reconstruction surgery for free for a young patient who had undergone a mastectomy for cancer. Spurred by this gap in patient care, his advocacy in New York State and then nationally led to the passage of the Women's Health and Cancer Rights Act in 1998 which not only guarantees coverage for breast reconstruction but also prohibits insurers from limiting hospital stays after mastectomies and requires coverage for treatment of lymphedema, leading to expanded access to reconstruction and contributing to decreases in disparities in reconstruction [5, 6].

My field of trauma surgery is replete with examples of surgeons using the insights gained from personal experiences and patient care. Dr. Joseph Sakran was inspired to become a trauma surgeon by his own experiences as a gunshot wound survivor and has become a powerful advocate for firearm injury prevention within and beyond the profession. Among other roles, he serves as the Board Chair and Chief Medical Officer of Brady United [7]. In 2022, this long-term collaboration contributed to the passage of the first federal firearms legislation in 30 years—the Safer Communities Act [8]. While this law did not address all facets of firearm safety reform that the U.S. needs, it made the most of the feasible opportunities to promote safety.

Working with the press is often essential to advocacy efforts, and developing the skills and connections to write for and speak to the public through op-eds and interviews can help us advance our goals. Dr. Jessica Beard is a trauma surgeon at Temple University who has taken this mission further. Based on her clinical experience and research [9–11] showing how cursory coverage of firearm injury can harm individuals and can hinder public understanding of the issue, she became determined to change the way that the media reports on gun violence and its victims. In collaboration with Jim MacMillan, Dr. Beard co-founded the Initiative for Better Gun Violence Reporting, leading to the establishment of the Philadelphia Center for Gun Violence Reporting, which has most recently led to the formation of the Association of Gun Violence Reporters, dedicated to making coverage more comprehensive and solutions-oriented [12].

Surgical Organizations

Our professional societies are key sites of advocacy for change within and beyond surgery. Of course, the American College of Surgeons is the largest and best-established convening body. The ACS can have a powerful voice to advocate for the issues that affect surgeons and surgeries, but by nature of its size, it contains a diversity of views that may limit the topics it can address that. At times, advocacy within the college can lead to policy changes that affect the field as a whole. Clinical subspecialty societies can advance the care of the patients they treat and can collaborate with patient groups or prevention efforts, as well.

Several organizations also convene surgeons on the basis of a minoritized identity within the field. Several identity or affinity-oriented surgical societies can also form a bridge, advocating both for surgeons within surgery and for surgeons within their workplaces, as well as for patients who experience exclusion, bias, or discrimination. The Association of Women in Surgery was founded in 1981 [13], and the Society of Black Academic Surgeons in 1987 [14], followed by the Society of Asian Academic Surgeons [15] in 2012 and the Latino Surgical Society in 2017 [16], and, most recently, the Native American Surgical Society in 2024 [17]. These organizations serve to connect members with shared experiences in life and in surgery, to provide representation, and to tackle shared challenges.

I have been fortunate to be part of the development of the Association for Out Surgeons and Allies (AOSA) since shortly after its founding by Dr. Nicole Goulet and colleagues in 2019 [18]. For me, AOSA represents how surgery mirrors, but also trails, our larger society. When I started medical school in 2007, I had been out as queer for a decade. I was immersed in queer community, and the ignorance and invisibility regarding LGBTQ+ people that I encountered in medical school was a shock. I didn't expect to become a leader of my medical school's LGBTQ+ group, but since there was only one other out student in my class of more than 250, the two of us took it on, focusing on basic awareness and education. There were scarcely any out faculty in any field, and I connected with the first queer surgeons I encountered primarily through their OR soundtracks. When it comes to LGBTQ+ people in surgery, representation is still primary. Simply seeing or knowing queer people in surgery is a victory that opens up our field to students and trainees who can see surgery as an option. With luck, this work opens up our field to become a place where LGBTQ+ surgeons can be themselves, and, by bringing their whole selves, create a richer and more open environment for everyone. AOSA helps with that, giving representation for LGBTQ+ people in surgery a home. As the organization becomes more established, we can extend beyond representation and mentorship to both providing education to programs and departments, as well as opportunities to our members and resources to our patients and communities.

Conclusion

There is nothing uniquely female about advocacy in surgery, but when I was invited to contribute a chapter on breaking barriers, I found myself thinking less of the barriers within surgery than the barriers that can separate surgery and surgeons from the rest of the world. In whatever way being women in surgery still makes us outsiders, perhaps we can use that positionality to grow our understanding of what surgery can be. But sometimes the pressures of just getting by within surgery can lock us into narrow views of success, so I go back to some of the privileges I mentioned at the beginning. The privilege of having the skills that can help another person heal already makes us successful. We are already here, and I hope we can continue to build on those fundamental successes to broaden our mission.

References

1. Social Determinants of Health 101 for Health Care: Five Plus Five—NAM. Accessed 7 June 2025. https://nam.edu/perspectives/social-determinants-of-health-101-for-health-care-five-plus-five/
2. Greenthal E, Jia J, Poblacion A, James T. Patient experiences and provider perspectives on a hospital-based food pantry: a mixed methods evaluation study. *Public Health Nutr.* 2019;22(17):3261-3269.https://doi.org/10.1017/S1368980019002040
3. Preventive Food Pantry. Boston Medical Center. Accessed 7 June 2025. https://www.bmc.org/nourishing-our-community/preventive-food-pantry

4. Corbisiero MF, Acker SN, Bothwell S, Christian N. Transforming Perceptions: The Impact of a Formal Parental Leave Policy on Surgical Trainees. *J Surg Educ*. 2024;81(6):816-822.https://doi.org/10.1016/j.jsurg.2024.03.007

5. Fisher MI. The Art and Science of Lymphedema Care. *Rehabilitation Oncology*. 2025;43(2):67.https://doi.org/10.1097/01.REO.0000000000000390

6. Rubenstein RN, Nelson JA, Azoury SC, et al. Disparity Reduction in U.S. Breast Reconstruction: An Analysis from 2005 to 2017 Using 3 Nationwide Data Sets. *Plast Reconstr Surg*. 2024;154(6):1065e-1075e.https://doi.org/10.1097/PRS.0000000000011432

7. Dr. Joseph Sakran. Brady United. Accessed 7 June 2025. https://www.bradyunited.org/about-us/our-team/experts/dr-joseph-sakran

8. Sen. Rubio M [R F. Text—S.2938—117th Congress (2021–2022): Bipartisan Safer Communities Act. June 25, 2022. Accessed 7 June 2025. https://www.congress.gov/bill/117th-congress/senate-bill/2938/text

9. Beard JH, Midberry J, Afif IN, Dauer E, MacMillan J, Jacoby SF. "Like I'm a nobody:" firearm-injured peoples' perspectives on news media reporting about firearm violence. *SSM—Qualitative Research in Health*. 2023;3:100212.https://doi.org/10.1016/j.ssmqr.2022.100212

10. Beard JH, Trombley S, Walker T, et al. Public health framing of firearm violence on local television news in Philadelphia, PA, USA: a quantitative content analysis. *BMC Public Health*. 2024;24(1):1221.https://doi.org/10.1186/s12889-024-18718-0

11. Beard JH, Eschliman EL, Wamakima A, Morrison CN, MacMillan J, Midberry J. Defining harmful news reporting on community firearm violence: A modified Delphi consensus study. *PLoS One*. 2024;19(12):e0316026. doi:https://doi.org/10.1371/journal.pone.0316026

12. Philadelphia Center For Gun Violence Reporting—Preventing harm by changing media narratives on gun violence. December 29, 2021. Accessed 7 June 2025. https://www.pcgvr.org/

13. American Women in Surgery (AWS). Accessed 7 June 2025. https://www.womensurgeons.org/about

14. The Society of Black Academic Surgeons (SBAS). Accessed 7 June 2025. http://www.sbas.net

15. The Society of Asian Academic Surgeons (SAAS). Accessed 7 June 2025. https://www.asian-surgeon.org/about/history/

16. Latino Surgical Society (LSS). Accessed 7 June 2025. https://www.latinosurgicalsociety.org/about

17. Native American Surgical Society (NASS). Accessed 7 June 2025. https://www.nativeamericansurgicalsociety.org

18. Association of Out Surgeons and Allies (AOSA). Accessed 7 June 2025. https://www.outsurgeons.org/

Part V

Innovations and Advancements in Surgery

Chapter 17
Emerging Technologies in Surgery

Vashti Bandy, Alyssa Habermann, Arunima Punjala,
and Kandace P. McGuire

Introduction

The field of surgery is rapidly driven by innovation, with the use of technology impacting the delivery, training, and planning for surgical procedures. In the last few decades, surgery has been transformed by minimally invasive techniques, advancements in imaging, and the use of artificial and nonhuman tissue implantation to expand care. As medicine continues to evolve, the applications of artificial intelligence (AI), virtual reality (VR), and three-dimensional (3D) printing show promise towards a future of improving surgical outcomes and minimizing risks for patients.

AI algorithms in medicine have been used to aid in diagnosis, but can now be utilized for preoperative planning, intraoperative decision-making, and predictions for surgical complications. VR's ability to allow for immersive simulation has transformed surgical training as novice surgeons can practice precision and technical dexterity prior to entering the operating room. Meanwhile, 3D printing has been able to individualize surgical procedures by creating patient-specific anatomical models and developing customized implants. Altogether, these technologies are not only augmenting surgical skills but also revolutionizing the efficiency and delivery of patient care. This chapter explores the current state of these emerging technologies in surgery to discuss their roles, future potential, and challenges in reshaping the field.

V. Bandy · A. Habermann · A. Punjala
Department of Surgery, Virginia Commonwealth University, Richmond, VA, USA
e-mail: vashti.bandy@vcuhealth.org; Alyssa.Habermann@vcuhealth.org;
arunima.punjala@vcuhealth.org

K. P. McGuire (✉)
Chief of Breast Surgery, Professor of Surgery, Department of Surgery,
Virginia Commonwealth University, Richmond, VA, USA
e-mail: kandace.mcguire@vcuhealth.org

K. Yoon-Flannery et al. (eds.), *Women in Surgery*,
https://doi.org/10.1007/978-3-032-10971-2_17

Artificial Intelligence

The origin of AI can be traced back to the 1956 Dartmouth Summer Research Project, where intellectuals first discussed the idea of machines replicating human intelligence. While the media fantasizes a world in which robots appear human-like and function independently, in reality, AI is limited to performing select and narrow tasks. Machine learning is a subfield of AI which encompasses neural networks and deep learning to enable computers to learn from datasets. In healthcare, machine learning algorithms have already transformed the ability to recommend diagnoses efficiently in specialties like radiology and pathology, where pattern recognition is imperative [11, 12, 35].

With advancements in technology, AI is a leading pathway through which surgeons can optimize care for their patients. Beginning with the preoperative phase, surgeons can utilize large datasets and advanced algorithms to improve risk stratification for patients considering surgery. Currently, an overwhelming number of risk calculators exist for specialists to assess a patient's fit for surgery; however, these calculations frequently underperform as they lack regional applicability and may rely on subjective assessments of preoperative health [4, 8, 11]. Tools such as the POTTER recognize that preoperative risk factors are not linear, and the interaction of comorbidities can weigh differently on outcomes. By combining inputs from the National Surgical Quality Improvement Program (NSQIP), machine-learning algorithms produced an AI-based decision tree that works to analyze patient histories, genetics, labs, and comorbidities to predict the likelihood of postoperative complications and outcomes in emergent surgeries [3]. Similar programs have been developed with excellent specificity and sensitivity for predicting results, such as Pythia or MySurgicalRisk score, which utilizes the electronic medical record at a single institution to combat the effects of local differences on care [4, 8]. With AI's ability to combine immense data into evidence-based predictions, surgeons are able to anticipate and mitigate risks and provide individualized counseling on postoperative expectations.

In the intraoperative phase, surgeons can utilize AI to provide real-time feedback and collaborate in informed critical decision-making. With the evolution of robotic surgery, AI algorithms improve instrument precision, enhance visualization, and can adjust dexterity to match each surgeon's specific needs. Merging videos of operations has already assisted general surgeons with highlighting critical views in invasive procedures. Visual cues alone can allow AI to make suggestions based on pattern recognition, object detection, and image processing of past footage [11]. This technology can guide and warn surgeons during difficult cases and has improved accuracy in surgeries such as cholecystectomy, sleeve gastrectomy, and sigmoidectomy [10, 13, 14]. Moreover, AI can be used to provide education by compiling hours of videos from a surgeon's prior operations into condensed and annotated segments of repeated patterns to provide technical critiques. This feedback can allow trainees to review their progress with an expert surgeon in the field to improve their acumen, much like how athletes improve by reviewing their performances on videotape with a coach [11, 35].

While the potential growth for AI in surgery is vast, its application in the field comes with significant challenges, particularly in the realm of data quality and ethics. AI's success largely relies on substantial quality and diverse data to train its algorithms. If these datasets are narrow, there is a high risk for bias in their recommendations [23]. Furthermore, while AI continues to learn from its inputs, understanding how much responsibility to delegate to machines remains controversial. The abilities gained from human expertise and experience are unmatched in providing depth to clinical judgement, but understanding the role of AI in decision-making is imperative for defining litigation and ongoing patient safety efforts [22]. As AI continues to advance, its ability to participate in patient care should be discussed so it can serve to augment patient outcomes with surgeon accountability.

The groundbreaking future for AI remains exciting with new considerations for the field of surgery. As AI machine learning algorithms improve, so will their integration into surgical practice. As surgeons and patients become more comfortable with incorporating its role in healthcare, this tool demonstrates promise for improving precision, efficiency, and safety for surgical procedures. With continued research, validation, and ethical considerations analyzed, AI is on its way to formidably transforming the future of surgical care.

Virtual/Augmented Reality

Virtual and augmented reality (VR and AR) have become essential to ongoing advancements in medicine. While both technologies are similar, VR creates a fully virtual environment while AR overlays digital elements—such as images, video frames, and 3D graphics—to enhance the real world. Initially developed for entertainment, VR and AR began entering the surgical field in the early 2000s. One notable example is AccuVein's AR glasses, developed in 2009, which provide a visual overlay of underlying veins on a patient's skin to assist with venipuncture—demonstrating technology's ability to improve surgical precision. Between 2016 and 2019, companies further expanded the use of VR and AR in surgical training by developing immersive training modules that allowed surgeons to practice procedures repeatedly in a risk-free environment. The COVID-19 pandemic then accelerated the adoption of these technologies, enabling innovative solutions for remote consultations, diagnostics, and surgeries [20, 33].

In the operating room, AR has shown significant potential to enhance treatment outcomes for technically complex cases by creating a hybrid patient model that blends real and virtual patient data. This hybrid model offers numerous benefits. By shifting data displays from 2D screens to the surgical field itself, AR allows surgeons to access critical information without diverting their eyes or hands from the operative area. This eliminates the need for multiple monitors displaying different aspects of patient data and improves safety and precision during procedures. A hybrid model can incorporate preoperative imaging—such as computed tomography (CT) and magnetic resonance imaging (MRI)—alongside intraoperative data and can even coordinate auditory or visual systems to ensure precise instrument tracking, whether moved directly by a surgeon or via a robotic system [7]. Furthermore, AR can superimpose 3D anatomical images of the target organ onto the operating field, essentially creating a 3D atlas. Neurosurgery, otolaryngology, and maxillofacial surgery have been early adopters of this technology, although its use is rapidly expanding into other specialties. In hepatobiliary surgery, a review of 28 studies performed between 2020 and 2022 involving 183 patients undergoing AR-assisted surgery evidenced greater resection margins and lower variability compared to the use of intraoperative ultrasonography [1]. In breast cancer surgery, AR visualization enables surgeons to perceive the exact 3D location of the tumor as if it were visible through the skin, maximizing breast conservation and reducing the risk of recurrence [26].

Beyond its ability to enhance surgical techniques and outcomes, AR is being explored for its potential to improve the patient experience through preoperative education. In a single-institution clinical trial, 95 patients were randomized to receive either traditional preoperative education with handouts or a preoperative interactive AR experience using an AR headset. The AR experience involved visually walking patients through their trip to the operating room, accompanied by narration from their surgeon. Study results demonstrated a significant decrease in anxiety from the initial screening to the perioperative survey in the AR group, with an effect that lasted up to the time of surgery. In contrast, the control group experienced an increase in anxiety [24]. Additional studies have explored the use of AR and VR in patient education to improve health literacy and patients' understanding of their disease process and treatment plans.

While the benefits of integrating AR and VR into surgical treatment are numerous—both realized and unexplored—there are also many challenges. A technical limitation for any surgeon in the AR environment is that the target organ does not always behave as expected. This issue is marked for pliable, intra-abdominal organs as opposed to more rigid structures such as the brain or bones. The widespread adoption of these technologies will also depend on financial incentives, supportive legislation, and collaboration with medical technology experts to ensure their safety and cost-effectiveness [29].

3D Printing

Over the past few decades, 3D printing has become increasingly prevalent within the field of surgery. It confers the advantage over traditional two-dimensional (2D) imaging modalities, such as computed tomography (CT) and magnetic resonance imaging (MRI), of providing improved visual and tactile interaction with patient-specific anatomy. Particularly, it allows for a better understanding of the spatial relationships between anatomical features. Its utilization can be broken down primarily into the following categories: presurgical planning models, advanced surgical planning and implants, trainee education models, and patient education models.

The process of creating a 3D model involves segmentation, printing, and post-processing. Segmentation refers to the use of computer software to create a digital model based on cross-sectional imaging. The delineation of different anatomical features is performed automatically by the software, with the opportunity for the user to make corrections based on their expertise. Once the virtual model is complete, printing can be performed using a variety of materials, such as metals and photopolymers with different colors and degrees of transparency, deformability, and strength. Lastly, post-processing is performed, during which any scaffolding and extra material are removed to finalize the model. Each step of the process is customizable, allowing for the creation of a model that fits a specific clinical need.

Presurgical planning refers to the creation of a 3D model as a visual and tactile aid for assistance in planning a surgical procedure. The field of orthopedic surgery was one of the early adopters of 3D models for presurgical planning, which have been well-studied and shown to reduce operative time and improve surgical accuracy and safety in spine, hip/pelvis, knee, and foot/ankle surgery [2]. Presurgical planning using 3D models has been similarly well-studied in urology, showing decreased estimated blood loss with their use in nephrectomy and lower positive margin rate with their use in prostatectomy [5, 18, 28]. In more recent years, the technology has been applied across a wide range of surgical specialties. In cardiac surgery, 3D models have been used to demonstrate coronary artery abnormalities, high-order coronary artery malformations, and primary cardiac tumors [27]. In thoracic surgery, 3D modeling has been used for tumor localization and planning of lung resection, and has been reported to reduce unnecessary removal of lung tissue and access injuries [15]. In vascular surgery, 3D models are especially useful for arterial aneurysms and can aid with appropriate graft selection [31]. In breast surgery, 3D models have been used for optimized tumor localization in breast conserving therapy and for accurate analysis of breast volume, shape, and contour preoperatively to allow for improved symmetry in breast reconstruction [9]. In hepatobiliary and pancreatic surgery, 3D printing has been incorporated into surgical planning for benign and malignant tumors [16, 30]. In esophagogastric surgery, 3D printing has proven helpful in generating a "vascular roadmap" for surgical guidance and is particularly useful in cases of anatomic variance; it has also been used for gastric cancer staging [25]. In colorectal surgery, there have been several prospective randomized controlled trials that have shown decreased blood loss and operative time with the use of 3D models for presurgical planning in colon and rectal cancer [6, 17].

Advanced surgical planning denotes the use of sterilized, patient-specific 3D printed objects in the intraoperative setting. This largely pertains to surgical guides and implants and to date has been most utilized in fields which work frequently with bone, such as orthopedic and maxillofacial surgery [19]. Examples include patient-specific plates in craniofacial surgery and pedicle screw templates in spine surgery. There is also the potential to create 3D-printed organs and soft tissues using biological scaffolding, but this technology is still in its infancy.

Three-dimensional printing holds great value within the realm of surgical education and can benefit learners of all levels. Educational models have been created for use by medical students and residents across virtually all surgical specialties and have 95% satisfaction rates among learners [32]. Advantages of using such models for education over 2D imaging include ability to visualize anatomy in actual 3D space, mimicking true-to-life anatomy, and the ability to rotate the model to understand spatial anatomy from various viewpoints. Similarly, 3D printing can be used to improve patient understanding of anatomy, disease processes, and planned interventions [34, 36] (Figs. 17.1, 17.2 and 17.3).

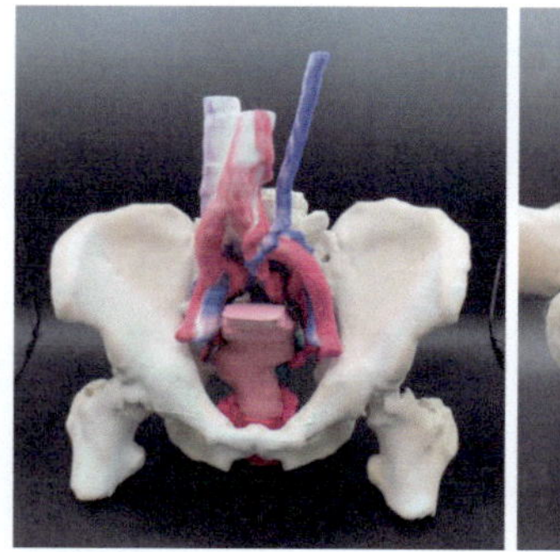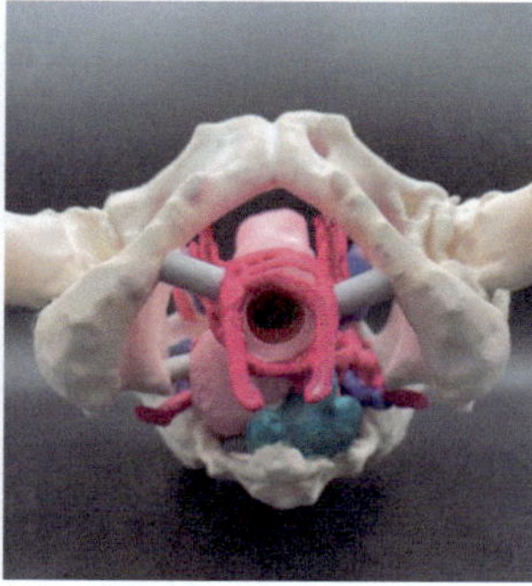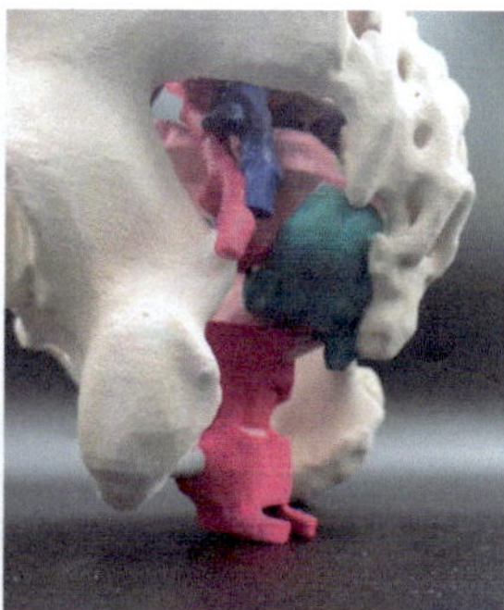

Fig. 17.1 3D-printed model of presacral tumor (green) with bone (beige), arteries (red), veins (blue), rectum (light pink), and levator ani/external anal sphincter muscles (dark pink)

Fig. 17.2 3D-printed model of sleeve gastrectomy converted to Roux-en-Y gastric bypass complicated by retained fundus. Bone is in beige, diaphragm in red, GI tract in clear, and staple line in blue

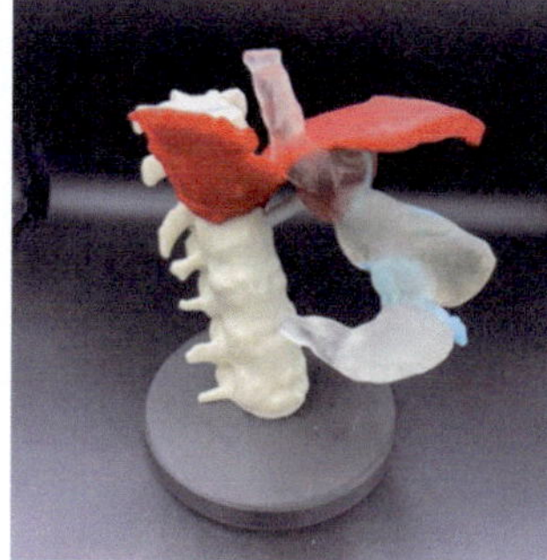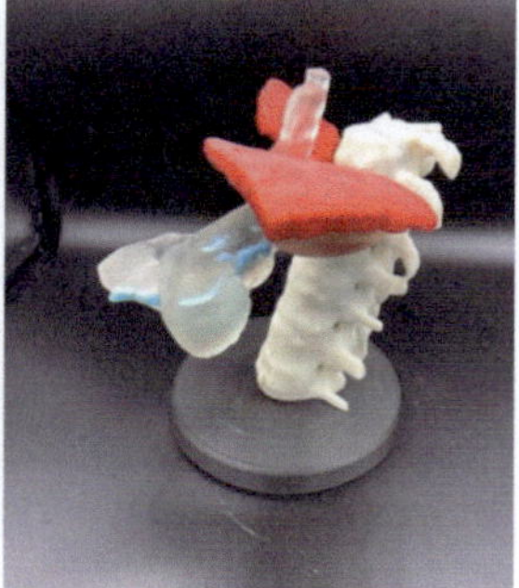

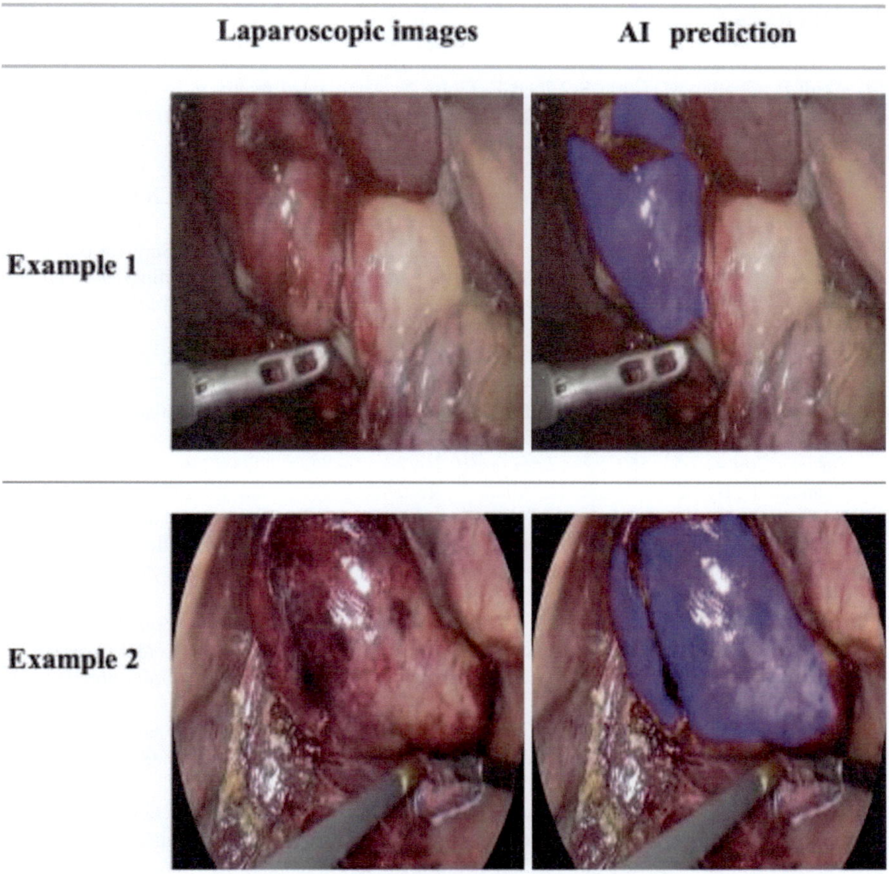

Laparoscopic images	**AI prediction**
Example 1	
Example 2	

Fig. 17.3 Use of AI to predict area of scarring (purple) during a laparoscopic cholecystectomy [21]

Conclusion

In the future, AI, VR, and 3D printing, along with many other surgical technologies, will continue to push the boundaries of medicine. As AI becomes more widespread, surgeons can hope for efficiency and improved safety in their practice. Virtual and augmented reality show promise to enhance surgical techniques and outcomes, while innovation and collaboration continue to shape their full potential in the operating room. 3D printing has been established to be useful in presurgical planning, advanced surgical planning, surgical trainee education, and patient education. We look forward to the more widespread use of these models as part of clinical practice, education, and ongoing development of patient-specific biologic organ and tissue models for implantation.

References

1. Acidi B, Ghallab M, Cotin S, Vibert E, Golse N. Augmented reality in liver surgery. *J Visc Surg.* 2023 Apr;160(2):118–126. https://doi.org/10.1016/j.jviscsurg.2023.01.008. Epub 2023 Feb 13. PMID: 36792394.

2. Alemayehu, D. G., Zhang, Z., Tahir, E., Gateau, D., Zhang, D.-F., & Ma, X. (2021). Preoperative Planning Using 3D Printing Technology in Orthopedic Surgery. *BioMed Research International*, *2021*(1), 7940242. https://doi.org/10.1155/2021/7940242

3. Bertsimas, D., Dunn, J., Velmahos, G. C., & Kaafarani, H. M. A. (2018). Surgical risk is not linear: Derivation and validation of a novel, user-friendly, and machine-learning-based predictive OPTIMal Trees in Emergency Surgery Risk (POTTER) calculator. *Annals of Surgery*, *268*(4), 574–583. https://doi.org/10.1097/sla.0000000000002956

4. Bihorac, A., Ozrazgat-Baslanti, T., Ebadi, A., Motaei, A., Madkour, M., Pardalos, P. M., Lipori, G., Hogan, W. R., Efron, P. A., Moore, F., Moldawer, L. L., Wang, D. Z., Hobson, C. E., Rashidi, P., Li, X., & Momcilovic, P. (2018). MySurgeryRisk: Development and validation of a machine-learning risk algorithm for major complications and death after surgery. *Annals of Surgery*, *269*(4), 652–662. https://doi.org/10.1097/sla.0000000000002706

5. Chandak, P., Byrne, N., Lynch, H., Allen, C., Rottenberg, G., Chandra, A., Raison, N., Ahmed, H., Kasivisvanathan, V., Elhage, O., & Dasgupta, P. (2018). Three-dimensional printing in robot-assisted radical prostatectomy—An Idea, Development, Exploration, Assessment, Long-term follow-up (IDEAL) Phase 2a study. *BJU International*, *122*(3), 360–361. https://doi.org/10.1111/bju.14189

6. Chen, Y., Bian, L., Zhou, H., Wu, D., Xu, J., Gu, C., Fan, X., Liu, Z., Zou, J., Xia, J., & Xu, Z. (2020). Usefulness of three-dimensional printing of superior mesenteric vessels in right hemicolon cancer surgery. *Scientific Reports*, *10*(1), Article 1. https://doi.org/10.1038/s41598-020-68578-y

7. Chopra H, Munjal K, Arora S, Bibi S, Biswas P. Role of augmented reality in surgery: editorial. *Int J Surg.* 2024 May 1;110(5):2526–2528. https://doi.org/10.1097/JS9.0000000000001219. PMID: 38363990; PMCID: PMC11093447.

8. Corey, K. M., Kashyap, S., Lorenzi, E., Lagoo-Deenadayalan, S. A., Heller, K., Whalen, K., Balu, S., Heflin, M. T., McDonald, S. R., Swaminathan, M., & Sendak, M. (2018). Development and validation of machine learning models to identify high-risk surgical patients using automatically curated electronic health record data (Pythia): A retrospective, single-site study. *PLoS Medicine*, *15*(11), e1002701. https://doi.org/10.1371/journal.pmed.1002701

9. Galstyan, A., Bunker, M. J., Lobo, F., Sims, R., Inziello, J., Stubbs, J., Mukhtar, R., & Kelil, T. (2021). Applications of 3D printing in breast cancer management. *3D Printing in Medicine*, *7*(1), 6. https://doi.org/10.1186/s41205-021-00095-8

10. Hashimoto, D. A., Rosman, G., Witkowski, E. R., Stafford, C., Navarette-Welton, A. J., Rattner, D. W., Lillemoe, K. D., Rus, D. L., & Meireles, O. R. (2019). Computer Vision analysis of intraoperative video. *Annals of Surgery*, *270*(3), 414–421. https://doi.org/10.1097/sla.0000000000003460

11. Hashimoto, D. A., Ward, T. M., & Meireles, O. R. (2020). The role of artificial intelligence in surgery. *Advances in Surgery*, *54*, 89–101. https://doi.org/10.1016/j.yasu.2020.05.010

12. Howard, J. (2019). Artificial intelligence: Implications for the future of work. *American Journal of Industrial Medicine*, *62*(11), 917–926. https://doi.org/10.1002/ajim.23037

13. Kannan, S., Yengera, G., Mutter, D., Marescaux, J., & Padoy, N. (2019). Future-State predicting LSTM for early surgery type recognition. *IEEE Transactions on Medical Imaging*, *39*(3), 556–566. https://doi.org/10.1109/tmi.2019.2931158

14. Kitaguchi, D., Takeshita, N., Matsuzaki, H., Takano, H., Owada, Y., Enomoto, T., Oda, T., Miura, H., Yamanashi, T., Watanabe, M., Sato, D., Sugomori, Y., Hara, S., & Ito, M. (2019). Real-time automatic surgical phase recognition in laparoscopic sigmoidectomy using the convolutional neural network-based deep learning approach. *Surgical Endoscopy*, *34*(11), 4924–4931. https://doi.org/10.1007/s00464-019-07281-0

15. Kwok, J. K. S., Lau, R. W. H., Zhao, Z.-R., Yu, P. S. Y., Ho, J. Y. K., Chow, S. C. Y., Wan, I. Y. P., & Ng, C. S. H. (2018). Multi-dimensional printing in thoracic surgery: Current and future applications. *Journal of Thoracic Disease, 10*(Suppl 6), S756–S763. https://doi.org/10.21037/jtd.2018.02.91

16. Lopez-Lopez, V., Robles-Campos, R., García-Calderon, D., Lang, H., Cugat, E., Jiménez-Galanes, S., Férnandez-Cebrian, J. M., Sánchez-Turrión, V., Fernández-Fernández, J. M., Barrera-Gómez, M. Á., de la Cruz, J., Lopez-Conesa, A., Brusadin, R., Gomez-Perez, B., & Parrilla-Paricio, P. (2021). Applicability of 3D-printed models in hepatobiliary surgey: Results from "LIV3DPRINT" multicenter study. *HPB, 23*(5), 675–684. https://doi.org/10.1016/j.hpb.2020.09.020

17. Lu, F., Qiu, L., Yu, P., Xu, D.-L., Miao, Y.-C., & Wang, G. (2023). Application of a three-dimensional printed pelvic model in laparoscopic radical resection of rectal cancer. *Frontiers in Oncology, 13*, 1195404. https://doi.org/10.3389/fonc.2023.1195404

18. Maddox, M. M., Feibus, A., Liu, J., Wang, J., Thomas, R., & Silberstein, J. L. (2018). 3D-printed soft-tissue physical models of renal malignancies for individualized surgical simulation: A feasibility study. *Journal of Robotic Surgery, 12*(1), 27–33. https://doi.org/10.1007/s11701-017-0680-6

19. Malik, H. H., Darwood, A. R. J., Shaunak, S., Kulatilake, P., El-Hilly, A. A., Mulki, O., & Baskaradas, A. (2015). Three-dimensional printing in surgery: A review of current surgical applications. *Journal of Surgical Research, 199*(2), 512–522. https://doi.org/10.1016/j.jss.2015.06.051

20. Nickel F, Cizmic A, Chand M. Telestration and Augmented Reality in Minimally Invasive Surgery: An Invaluable Tool in the Age of COVID-19 for Remote Proctoring and Telementoring. *JAMA Surg.* 2022 Feb 1;157(2):169–170. https://doi.org/10.1001/jamasurg.2021.3604. PMID: 34705030

21. Orimoto H, Hirashita T, Ikeda S, Amano S, Kawamura M, Kawano Y, Takayama H, Masuda T, Endo Y, Matsunobu Y, Shinozuka K, Tokuyasu T, Inomata M. Development of an artificial intelligence system to indicate intraoperative findings of scarring in laparoscopic cholecystectomy for cholecystitis. Surg Endosc. 2025 Feb;39(2):1379–1387. https://doi.org/10.1007/s00464-024-11514-2. Epub 2025 Jan 21. PMID: 39838147; PMCID: PMC11794413.

22. O'Sullivan, S., Nevejans, N., Allen, C., Blyth, A., Leonard, S., Pagallo, U., Holzinger, K., Holzinger, A., Sajid, M. I., & Ashrafian, H. (2018). Legal, regulatory, and ethical frameworks for development of standards in artificial intelligence (AI) and autonomous robotic surgery. *International Journal of Medical Robotics and Computer Assisted Surgery, 15*(1). https://doi.org/10.1002/rcs.1968

23. Panch, T., Mattie, H., & Atun, R. (2019). Artificial intelligence and algorithmic bias: implications for health systems. *Journal of Global Health, 9*(2). https://doi.org/10.7189/jogh.09.020318

24. Rizzo MG Jr, Costello JP 2nd, Luxenburg D, Cohen JL, Alberti N, Kaplan LD. Augmented Reality for Perioperative Anxiety in Patients Undergoing Surgery: A Randomized Clinical Trial. *JAMA Netw Open.* 2023 Aug 1;6(8):e2329310. https://doi.org/10.1001/jamanetworkopen.2023.29310. PMID: 37589975; PMCID: PMC10436133.

25. Robb, H., Scrimgeour, G., Boshier, P., Przedlacka, A., Balyasnikova, S., Brown, G., Bello, F., & Kontovounisios, C. (2022). The current and possible future role of 3D modelling within oesophagogastric surgery: A scoping review. *Surgical Endoscopy, 36*(8), 5907–5920. https://doi.org/10.1007/s00464-022-09176-z

26. Sato Y, Nakamoto M, Tamaki Y, et al. Image guidance of breast cancer surgery using 3-D ultrasound images and augmented reality visualization. IEEE Trans Med Imaging. 1998;17:681–693.

27. Shabbak, A., Masoumkhani, F., Fallah, A., Amani-Beni, R., Mohammadpour, H., Shahbazi, T., & Bakhshi, A. (2024). 3D Printing for Cardiovascular Surgery and Intervention: A Review Article. *Current Problems in Cardiology, 49*(1, Part B), 102086. https://doi.org/10.1016/j.cpcardiol.2023.102086

28. Shin, T., Ukimura, O., & Gill, I. S. (2016). Three-dimensional Printed Model of Prostate Anatomy and Targeted Biopsy-proven Index Tumor to Facilitate Nerve-sparing Prostatectomy. *European Urology, 69*(2), 377–379. https://doi.org/10.1016/j.eururo.2015.09.024

29. Shuhaiber JH. Augmented reality in surgery. Arch Surg. 2004 Feb;139(2):170–4. https://doi.org/10.1001/archsurg.139.2.170.

30. Song, C., Min, J. H., Jeong, W. K., Kim, S. H., Heo, J. S., Han, I. W., Shin, S. H., Yoon, S. J., Choi, S.-Y., & Moon, S. (2023). Use of individualized 3D-printed models of pancreatic cancer to improve surgeons' anatomic understanding and surgical planning. *European Radiology, 33*(11), 7646–7655. https://doi.org/10.1007/s00330-023-09756-0

31. Tam, C. H. A., Chan, Y. C., Law, Y., & Cheng, S. W. K. (2018). The Role of Three- Dimensional Printing in Contemporary Vascular and Endovascular Surgery: A Systematic Review. *Annals of Vascular Surgery, 53*, 243–254. https://doi.org/10.1016/j.avsg.2018.04.038

32. Taritsa, I. C., Lee, D., Foppiani, J., Escobar, M. J., Alvarez, A. H., Schuster, K. A., Lin, S. J., & Lee, B. T. (2024). Three-Dimensional Printing in Surgical Education: An Updated Systematic Review of the Literature. *Journal of Surgical Research, 300*, 425–431. https://doi.org/10.1016/j.jss.2024.04.077

33. VR & AR in the healthcare domain: A timeline. PROVEN Reality. (2024, September 1). https://provenreality.com/vr-ar-in-the-healthcare-domain-a-timeline/

34. Wake, N., Rosenkrantz, A. B., Huang, R., Park, K. U., Wysock, J. S., Taneja, S. S., Huang, W. C., Sodickson, D. K., & Chandarana, H. (2019). Patient-specific 3D printed and augmented reality kidney and prostate cancer models: Impact on patient education. *3D Printing in Medicine, 5*(1), 4. https://doi.org/10.1186/s41205-019-0041-3

35. Ward, T. M., Mascagni, P., Madani, A., Padoy, N., Perretta, S., & Hashimoto, D. A. (2021). Surgical data science and artificial intelligence for surgical education. *Journal of Surgical Oncology, 124*(2), 221–230. https://doi.org/10.1002/jso.26496

36. Zhuang, Y., Zhou, M., Liu, S., Wu, J., Wang, R., & Chen, C. (2019). Effectiveness of personalized 3D printed models for patient education in degenerative lumbar disease. *Patient Education and Counseling, 102*(10), 1875–1881. https://doi.org/10.1016/j.pec.2019.05.006

Chapter 18
Embracing Robotics and Minimally Invasive Techniques, Advancing the Field as a Woman in Surgery

Andrea Pakula

Introduction

My journey into robotic surgery began when I was a new Trauma and Critical Care attending. It may seem strange to hear those two areas of surgery in the same sentence, and many people thought the same, so I'll try to explain how this all came about.

There are key people in my life, both male and female, who played an integral part in not only my adoption of robotic surgery but also the evolution of my career. Their support of me, and others like me, has contributed greatly to women being more equally represented in surgery and on panels of many society meetings. I would like to dedicate this chapter to those who believed in me. I would not be where I am today without their support and encouragement.

During my residency and fellowship training, I had no exposure to robotic-assisted surgery. My Chair of Surgery during my residency, Dr. Maureen Martin, was insistent on me finding a "niche" outside of Trauma and Critical Care, as things were beginning to become more nonoperative in Trauma. It was early in my training that I developed a strong interest in abdominal wall anatomy and reconstructive surgeries for complex hernias. My Trauma Medical Director (TMD) at the time, Dr. Ruby Skinner, also had a strong interest in this area, which afforded me many opportunities to scrub in on a wide variety of hernia procedures. After I completed my Surgical Critical Care fellowship at the Mayo Clinic in Rochester, MN, I returned to my general residency program as an attending and joined the TMD, not only to grow the Trauma and ICU program, but also to build a practice around hernia and abdominal wall reconstruction.

A. Pakula (✉)
Department of Surgery, General, Bariatric and Hernia Surgery, Trauma, Critical Care and Acute Care Surgery, Adventist Health, Roseville, CA, USA
e-mail: apakula333@aol.com

K. Yoon-Flannery et al. (eds.), *Women in Surgery*,
https://doi.org/10.1007/978-3-032-10971-2_18

"

During my first year as a new attending, I participated in every course and hernia meeting that I could with the intention of improving my skillset and understanding of hernia and abdominal wall anatomy. At that time, I was operating primarily open with some laparoscopic techniques for hernia repair. Two years later, in 2016, a new Urology group was hired to the hospital, and with them came a da Vinci Xi Robotic Surgery Platform. I'd seen some podium talks about robotic-assisted surgery in hernia repair at the meetings, but it was not yet standard. I saw this as an opportunity for us to expand upon what we were offering to our hernia patients, so I asked my Chair to allow me to train. She supported the idea, and my TMD and I began our da Vinci training.

It was during my initial robotic training that I met a now very good friend, Dr. David Lourié. I had the opportunity to observe him perform da Vinci procedures in his operating room, and he later came to our hospital to proctor my first cases. He became an invaluable resource, not only for robotic technical advice but also for career advice.

Most general surgeons can hone their robotic skills with elective "bread and butter" cases such as gallbladders and small hernias. As trauma and acute care surgeons, we didn't have robust elective practices outside of complex hernias. Our learning curve was unique because our "bread and butter" cases were the acute gallbladders, appendectomies, and small hernias that presented to the emergency department with incarceration or strangulation. Due to the unpredictability of these types of cases, we spent a significant amount of time on the simulator to get as many touches as possible and gain familiarity and muscle memory with the technology.

If you've ever played a sport or a musical instrument, you know that mastering a new skill requires thousands of reps. With that in mind, I dedicated my practice to applying da Vinci surgery to every case I could during the first 4 months. This afforded me a broad base of experience, which led to my learning complex abdominal wall reconstruction techniques utilizing the robot, specifically transversus abdominis release or RoboTAR.

I attended a course specifically teaching RoboTAR, which was led by Dr. Conrad Ballecer and other experts in AWR and robotic surgery. It was inspirational, to say the least. Dr. Ballecer was then kind enough to come to California to proctor my first robotic TAR. This experience is what led me to recognize the value of being able to apply MIS surgery to not only the complex hernia patients, but also the acute care patients. There were numerous benefits to them not having a laparotomy, and I was happy to be able to offer this higher level of care and to begin to narrow the gap of health inequity for patients undergoing emergency surgery.

Less than a year into my robotic surgery experience, I attended a hernia meeting where my now very good friend, Conrad, was also in attendance. By this time, he had become one of my mentors for robotic abdominal wall reconstruction. After the meeting, he shared that he had recommended me as a speaker for one of the biggest robotic surgery conferences of the year, the Intuitive Connect meeting. Conrad saw something in me and pushed for me to be a part of the meeting. Not only to talk about my experience with robotic surgery, but also how I was applying it to Acute Care Surgery.

In 2018, I attended the Connect meeting, but only as an observer, not as faculty. The entire conference was predominantly led by male surgeons, all very good and well respected in the field, but as was so often the case at that time, very few female surgeons were on stage. This wasn't surprising, but it was disappointing. In that moment, I was determined to be on stage the following year. I became heavily involved with Intuitive Surgical and began teaching, proctoring, and doing local dinner presentations about my experience with da Vinci surgery from the perspective of a trauma and acute care surgeon. I began to put myself out there, actively posting my various surgeries and techniques on closed Facebook groups such as the International Hernia Collaboration and The Robotic Surgery Collaborative. It was with this exposure that I began to be recognized as an expert in the field of hernia, as well as robotic surgery. In 2019, I took the stage at Connect for the first time and am honored to have been a faculty member every year since. I am also happy to say that the number of female surgeons presenting and now leading that meeting, and many other meetings, increases each year.

My experience with robotic surgery continued to grow, and my application of the technology also grew. I was performing not only hernia and abdominal wall reconstruction surgeries, but was also performing increasingly more complex emergency procedures. However, like most hospitals at the time, robotic surgery at my hospital was only being performed during "regular business hours." We didn't have access to perform robotic surgery after hours or on weekends. This began my push for 24/7 access. As acute care surgeons, we don't have the luxury of scheduling our surgeries. Our patients come into the emergency department at any time of day and on any day of the week. I truly believe that every patient deserves the same level of care regardless of the time of day, and for acute care surgeons, especially, da Vinci has allowed us to minimize open surgery for our patients. By collaborating with the hospital administration and Intuitive, we were able to achieve expanded access and offer da Vinci surgery 24/7.

In 2020, I was recruited to a new hospital to help build their robotics program from the ground up. Over the next few years, through partnership and shared vision with a very supportive administrative team, we built a successful robotic surgery program, offering multispecialty robotic surgery and 24/7 access to patients.

At this point, I had stopped taking trauma call and put all of my energy into developing my practice in general surgery with a focus on hernia repair and abdominal wall reconstruction, and emergency general surgery. I also wanted to do my part in helping to advance the field of ACS, since it has always been based on open maximally invasive surgery. I began speaking more about my experiences with da Vinci ACS surgery, proctoring, and hosting surgeons in my operating room. I partnered with a friend and colleague, Dr. Matthew Martin, in starting a Minimally Invasive committee for one of the major trauma societies, and to this day, a robotic ACS course is held and filled annually. Acute Care Robotic surgery is now one of the largest growing areas of minimally invasive surgery in the United States, and it is because of this that we are able to continue to improve the equitable care that we deliver to our patients.

Conclusion

Whether you're a surgeon in academics or community-based practice, there are always opportunities for growth, but I strongly believe that to grow, you have to put yourself out there. What I've learned over the past 12 years of my career is that the early focus should be on becoming the best surgeon you can be. Not the best female surgeon, but the best surgeon. Women in medicine have faced additional barriers compared to our male counterparts, and I feel that one of the ways to address with this is to move forward as if those barriers don't exist. I've worked hard to develop my skills. I put myself out there for those skills to be recognized, and this is true for many women in the field. Although some of these gender biases do still exist, there's good news in that this is changing. There is increasing recruitment of women into the field of surgery, and for the past several years, more than 50% of medical students are women [1]. There are now many women rising to leadership positions in surgery, academics, and surgical societies [2].

Women in medicine need to continue to support and elevate each other, and male colleagues can also play an important role as mentors, providing career advice and helping to lead women into leadership positions and onto the podium as well [3].

I am thankful to be practicing during this time of incredible technological advancements and growing equality for female surgeons. I am truly grateful to those who have supported, encouraged, and believed in me.

References

1. Stephens EH, Heisler CA, Temkin SM, Miller P. 2020 The Current Status of Women in Surgery: How to Affect the Future JAMA Surg. 155(9):876–885
2. Pories SE, Turner PL, Greenberg CC, Babu MA, Parangi S. 2019 Leadership in American Surgery: Women are Risking to the Top. Ann Surg. 269(2):199–205
3. Wood DE. 2021 How can men be good allies for women in surgery? #HeForShe. J Thorac Dis. 13(1):492–501.

Chapter 19
Research and Development in Surgical Practices

Michelle C. Salazar and Katherine D. Gray

Research and development (R&D) in surgery is fundamental to advancing medical care, improving patient outcomes, and shaping the world of surgery as we know it. Over the centuries, innovations in surgery—from the development of anesthesia to that of robotic surgery—have transformed the field [8]. These advancements, however, have not been the result of isolated efforts but rather the product of collaboration in research and technological breakthroughs. Ultimately, the consequence of an essential feedback loop between science and clinical practice.

Women have played vital roles in driving innovation and progress in surgical R&D. Female surgeons' contributions to the field have been particularly evident in maternal and reproductive health, pediatric surgery, surgical education, and the development of safety protocols in surgery, but are notable throughout the surgical specialties [21]. By driving surgical R&D, women have helped ensure that surgery continues to evolve into a more technically advanced discipline, but also more inclusive, and ultimately more attuned to the diverse population it serves.

This chapter explores the contributions of women to surgical R&D, their unique perspectives, and the challenges they face in continuing to promote innovation in surgery.

The journey to becoming surgeons has been a challenging one for women. Although there are reports of ancient civilizations in Mesopotamia, Egypt, and Greece having had prominent female surgeons, the Middle Ages brought countless rulings and laws that barred women from practicing surgery [16]. Yet, women persisted. Such was the case of Dr. Miranda Stewart (1795–1865), who practiced surgery under the disguise of "Dr. James Barry," joined the army as a surgeon during the Napoleonic wars and eventually performed one of the first successful cesarean sections in 1820. She would only be discovered to be a woman upon her death [21].

M. C. Salazar · K. D. Gray (✉)
Memorial Sloan Kettering Cancer Center, New York, NY, USA
e-mail: salazarm@mskcc.org; grayk@mskcc.org

K. Yoon-Flannery et al. (eds.), *Women in Surgery*,
https://doi.org/10.1007/978-3-032-10971-2_19

In the United States, the challenges were no less. Dr. Elizabeth Blackwell, the first female physician, would not graduate until 1849. Unfortunately, she was not allowed to pursue her dream of becoming a surgeon as she was not granted a residency position despite graduating with honors. She would eventually open the Women's Medical College of New York [14]. Dr. Mary Edwards Walker graduated as the second female physician in the USA in 1855. After several years of practice as a surgical nurse, she would become the first female surgeon in the U.S. Army in 1863. Her service during the Civil War would be recognized with the Congressional Medal of Honor in 1865. To this day, she remains the only female to have been awarded this high distinction [1].

The landscape of surgery began to shift as medical education became more accessible to women in the USA. The 1970s would mark the beginning of this era. Propelled by the women's movement and key civil rights victories of the 1960s, women applied and entered medical schools in larger numbers than before [21]. Almost 50 years later, the percentage of women physicians in the USA has increased from 5% in 1970 to 38% in 2022 [5]. Although this effect has lagged in most surgical specialties, the current data points toward an ongoing increase in the percentage of female surgeons, with women making up 48% of general surgery residents in 2022 [6].

As more women have entered the field of surgery, many have driven advancements across various specialties. Notable examples include Dr. Alma Dea Morani, who used her background in art to fine-tune her passion for surgery, allowing her to become the first woman to be a plastic surgeon in the USA. She would establish the first Hand Surgery Clinic in Philadelphia in 1948, and one of the first in the USA [19]. Dr. Nina Starr Braunwald, a pioneer in the male-dominated field of cardiothoracic surgery, after years of research, in 1960, performed the first human mitral valve replacement using a valve of her own design [18]. Furthermore, Dr. Olga Jonasson, a transplant surgeon with an extensive research background in immunohistochemistry and immunobiology, who would complete the first kidney transplantation in Illinois in 1969 and who would become the first woman in the USA to be the Chair of an academic surgery department at Ohio State University in 1987[10].

Women have had a profound impact on several key areas of surgical practice, particularly in promoting women's health, improving pediatric surgery, and advancing surgical education. In the realm of women's health, female surgeons established some of the first screening centers for uterine cancer, were fierce advocates for birth control, and developed databases for breast cancer research [7, 17]. In pediatric surgery, women innovated in several areas, including using jeweler's instruments to perform surgery on small infants, describing the use of water-soluble contrast enemas to relieve uncomplicated meconium ileus, and describing the effects of the Mullerian Inhibiting Substance on congenital anomalies and cancer, amongst many others [13]. In surgical education, women have pioneered new models for training the next generation, including the development of new technology for surgical simulation as well as new ways of assessing competency of surgical skills [12]. Furthermore, women have been at the forefront of mentorship, recognizing its importance for the recruitment and retention of not only women but surgeons across the board. They have created networks and driven many initiatives at the level of associations such as the Association of Women Surgeons and the American College of Surgeons that provide guidance, encouragement, and professional development to aspiring female surgeons.

Despite the growing number of women entering the field of surgery and their substantial contributions, gender disparities remain a challenge, particularly in academic surgery. Since 2017, women have represented 50% or more of the medical students, and yet, only 13.5% of full professors of surgery are women [2]. Women also continue to encounter obstacles in ascending to leadership positions within academic surgery, with only 6.2% of them being division chiefs or department heads vs. 13.6% of their male surgeons in academia [20]. These disparities are further reflected in publication rates and citations, with women often underrepresented as lead and senior authors in top-tier surgical journals [4, 11]. Not surprisingly, even with female surgeon scientist obtaining their first NIH grant earlier in their careers and being as likely to obtain large-dollar grants as their male counterparts, they remain less likely to hold $750,000 or more in annual research funding [15]. Even with their substantial contributions, women in surgery are still fighting for equal recognition and resources to succeed in the world of academic surgery.

However, there are growing opportunities to address these challenges. Increasing focus on mentoring young female surgeons will help ensure that the next generation of women surgeon scientists is well-equipped to navigate the complexities of academic careers. Initiatives, like the mentorship network organized by the Association of Women Surgeons; research fellowships specifically targeting female scholars like the Nina Starr Braunwald Research Fellowship by the Thoracic Surgery Foundation; and institutional efforts to promote gender equity in the advancement of academic careers as well as to narrow the pay gap, have the potential of making a big difference [3]. Ultimately, the goal is not only to retain talented women in surgery but also to guarantee they have the tools to thrive in research and academic positions [9]. This will ensure that women continue to have a lasting impact in the world of surgery.

In conclusion, the contributions of women to research and development in surgery are undeniable. Female surgeons have not only achieved groundbreaking advancements in surgical techniques, education, research, and patient care, but they have also done so while having to overcome historical barriers. Despite these accomplishments, significant gender disparity still exists, particularly in leadership positions, research funding, and overall academic advancement. To fully realize the potential of women in surgery, it is crucial to address these challenges through mentorship, institutional support, and ongoing efforts to promote gender equity. Their success will allow the next generation of women surgeons to shape the future of surgery with even greater impact and innovation.

References

1. Alexander, K. L., Rothberg, E. Z. . (2023). *Mary Edwards Walker*. Retrieved 3/28/2025 from https://www.womenshistory.org/education-resources/biographies/mary-edwards-walker
2. Arya, S., Franco-Mesa, C., & Erben, Y. (2022). An analysis of gender disparities amongst United States medical students, general surgery residents, vascular surgery trainees, and the vascular surgery workforce. *Journal of Vascular Surgery, 75*(1), 5-9. https://doi.org/10.1016/j.jvs.2021.09.029
3. Association of Women Surgeons Awards. (2024). Retrieved 03/28/2025 from https://www.womensurgeons.org/awards
4. Bernardi, K., Lyons, N. B., Huang, L., Holihan, J. L., Olavarria, O. A., Loor, M. M., Ko, T. C., & Liang, M. K. (2020). Gender Disparity Among Surgical Peer-Reviewed Literature. *Journal of Surgical Research, 248*, 117-122. https://doi.org/10.1016/j.jss.2019.11.007
5. Boyle, P. D., Mi.; Kelly, R.; Nouri, Z. (2024). *Women Are Changing the Face of Medicine in America*. Retrieved 3/27/2025 from https://www.aamc.org/news/women-are-changing-face-medicine-america
6. Brotherton, S. E., & Etzel, S. I. (2023). Graduate Medical Education, 2022–2023. *JAMA, 330*(10), 988–1011. https://doi.org/10.1001/jama.2023.15520
7. Catharine MacFarlane. (2023). Retrieved 03/27/2025 from https://www.amwa-doc.org/awards/blackwell-exhibit/catharine-macfarlane-md/
8. Gawande, A. (2012). Two hundred years of surgery. *N Engl J Med, 366*(18), 1716–1723. https://doi.org/10.1056/NEJMra1202392
9. Greenup, R. A., & Pitt, S. C. (2020). Women in Academic Surgery: A Double-Edged Scalpel. *Acad Med, 95*(10), 1483–1484. https://doi.org/10.1097/acm.0000000000003592
10. Husser, W., & Neumayer, L. (2006). Olga Jonasson, MD: Surgeon, Mentor, Teacher, Friend. *Annals of Surgery, 244*(6), 839–840. https://doi.org/10.1097/01.sla.0000248100.13289.c0
11. Kane, W. J., Hedrick, T. L., & Schroen, A. T. (2022). Gender Disparity in the Citation of Surgical Research. *J Am Coll Surg, 234*(4), 624–631. https://doi.org/10.1097/xcs.0000000000000089
12. Medical Training Reinvented With the Help of a Woman's Touch. Retrieved 03/26/2025 from https://www.nibib.nih.gov/science-education/meet-a-scientist/carla-pugh-md-phd
13. Nakayama, D. K. (2018). Pioneering women in American pediatric surgery. *Journal of Pediatric Surgery, 53*(11), 2361–2368. https://doi.org/10.1016/j.jpedsurg.2018.08.038
14. Nallamotu, S., Vankayalapati, A., & Paruchuri, S. (2024). Dr. Elizabeth Blackwell (1821–1910): Opening Doors to Women in Medicine. *Cureus, 16*(10), e71899. https://doi.org/10.7759/cureus.71899
15. Nguyen, M., Gonzalez, L., Chaudhry, S. I., Ahuja, N., Pomahac, B., Newman, A., Cannon, A., Zarebski, S. A., Dardik, A., & Boatright, D. (2023). Gender Disparity in National Institutes of Health Funding Among Surgeon-Scientists From 1995 to 2020. *JAMA Netw Open, 6*(3), e233630. https://doi.org/10.1001/jamanetworkopen.2023.3630
16. Pastena, J. A. (1993). Women in Surgery: An Ancient Tradition. *Archives of Surgery, 128*(6), 622–626. https://doi.org/10.1001/archsurg.1993.01420180020004
17. Petro, J. (2023). *Remembering Dr. Susan Love (1949–2023)*. Retrieved 03/28/2025 from https://www.amwa-doc.org/news/remembering-dr-susan-love-1949-2023/
18. Singh, S., DiGiacomo, J. C., & Angus, L. D. G. (2021). "It Will Work": The Story of Nina Starr Braunwald and the First Successful Mitral Valve Replacement. *Ann Thorac Surg, 112*(3), 1023–1028. https://doi.org/10.1016/j.athoracsur.2021.03.096
19. Solomon, M. P., & Granick, M. S. (1997). Alma Dea Morani, MD: a pioneer in plastic surgery. *Ann Plast Surg, 38*(4), 431–436. https://doi.org/10.1097/00000637-199704000-00021

20. Valsangkar, N., Fecher, A. M., Rozycki, G. S., Blanton, C., Bell, T. M., Freischlag, J., Ahuja, N., Zimmers, T. A., & Koniaris, L. G. (2016). Understanding the Barriers to Hiring and Promoting Women in Surgical Subspecialties. *Journal of the American College of Surgeons, 223*(2). https://journals.lww.com/journalacs/fulltext/2016/08000/understanding_the_barriers_to_hiring_and_promoting.21.aspx
21. Wirtzfeld, D. A. (2009). The history of women in surgery. *Can J Surg, 52*(4), 317–320.

Chapter 20
Women Leading the Way in Surgical Innovation

Rachel M. Russo and Tandis Soltani

Introduction

> If girls were as exposed to female inventors as boys are to male inventors in their childhood communities, the gender gap in innovation would be half its current size [2].

Women surgeons are experts at turning obstacles into opportunities. The necessity of daily problem-solving has turned many women into natural innovators. Nonetheless, few women surgeons enter the surgical innovation space, and even fewer successfully navigate the journey of bringing a product to the marketplace. This chapter will explore the landscape of women in surgical innovation, explain why female surgeons should engage in innovation, and highlight lessons we have learned from women who are paving the way.

The Past

In 1977, *The Journal of the Royal College of General Practitioners* published an article titled "Doctors' Attitudes to Women in Medicine." The authors expressed a "moderate enthusiasm" within the medical profession for increasing the number of women doctors. However, they noted a "poorly organized and minimally supported

R. M. Russo (✉)
Department of General Surgery, Division of Acute Care Surgery, UC Davis Health, Sacramento, CA, USA
e-mail: rachelmrusso@gmail.com

T. Soltani
Assistant Professor of Surgery, Division of Acute Care Surgery and Surgical Critical Care, Department of Surgery, Loma Linda University Health, Loma Linda, CA, USA
e-mail: soltanitandis@gmail.com

K. Yoon-Flannery et al. (eds.), *Women in Surgery*,
https://doi.org/10.1007/978-3-032-10971-2_20

attempt" to balance domestic life with a professional career. They concluded that "until a more positive attitude develops within the profession, women doctors will not feel accepted as equals" [7].

The Present

Nearly 50 years later, these attitudes have been slow to change, especially in the field of surgical science. The surgical innovation sector continues to exhibit a significant gender disparity. In 2010, only one-quarter of the biomedical patents filed in the USA were held by women—3014 in total. This number still lags behind the 3347 patents filed by men in 1976, the first year that patent data became text-searchable. Although there has been some growth, with patents filed by women inventors increasing from roughly 6.3–16.2%, these figures still fall significantly short of equal representation [5].

The lack of gender parity in surgical technology and biotech is reflective of the lack of gender representation in surgery. Surgical training is long and challenging, with many women leaving the field at various stages. Although female medical students have outnumbered their male counterparts for three consecutive years, women represent only 38.1% of the active physician workforce in the United States and a mere 24.9% of general surgeons [11]. Furthermore, women hold an even smaller percentage of surgical leadership positions [8]. With fewer women leading surgical departments, fewer female surgeons attain the support necessary to dedicate time to surgical innovation.

When women work under women leaders, they benefit from a supportive environment that promotes authenticity, agency, and professional growth. Female department chairs create opportunities for other women to make significant contributions to advancements in health and science [5, 10]. Women innovators often focus on issues related to women's health, with the potential to advance health equity. A study of the U.S. Patent and Trademark Office (USPTO) databases identified 1551 unique female inventors who had patents for handheld surgical instruments or tools; many of these were designed for obstetric surgery or breast surgery or aimed to enhance the safety and ergonomics of existing devices, making them more suitable for women [12]. Although these innovations primarily aimed to improve women's health, many also positively affected care for all patients. However, these patents were much less likely to receive venture capital funding. While the "gender gap in innovation" is narrowing, it is estimated that it will take another 118 years to close completely [2].

Together, we have the power to change these odds. Every woman who enters the field of surgical innovation brings us all one step closer to better health and a more equitable work environment.

The Future

You have already taken the first step toward creating a better future for female innovators by becoming informed and, hopefully, inspired. Though women are underrepresented in surgery, in innovation, and even more so in surgical innovation, there has been progress. There are countless incredible women actively innovating, breaking barriers, and paving the way for your next step in translational science. We highlighted a few contemporaries (Drs. Katherine S. Blevins, MD, PhD; Melina R. Kibbe, MD; Rachel Russo, MD, MS; Sabina Siddiqui, MD; and Lee Wilke, MD) in our previous work [9]. We have summarized their advice to help you succeed in your surgical innovation journey:

- Always start by identifying a clinical need

  - Too often, innovators start backward, first developing a product and then searching for a suitable application for it
  - Only 3% of patents ever turn a profit [1, 3]. These odds can be enhanced by first identifying a need through customer discovery, analyzing the market, and recognizing stakeholders who will be pivotal to clinical adoption.

- Identify your allies

  - Assembling a strong team is crucial for success. It is far easier to join a successful team of innovators than to undertake the journey alone.
  - Learn the process, expand your social network, foster productive collaborations, and identify allies who will support you as you prepare to launch your own innovation.

- Use your resources

  - Most universities have a technology transfer office that can assist throughout the innovation process.
  - Regulatory consultants make their living by guiding innovators through the intricate maze of the Food and Drug Administration.
  - The National Institutes of Health has established Clinical Translational Science Award Programs at 60 leading medical institutions to provide coursework, advising, mentoring, and support for innovators at all stages of the process.

- Persevere!

  - Don't be discouraged if your first attempt isn't successful. Many great products cannot pass through the "valley of death"—the term for transitioning from the research lab to the consumer market.
  - Successful clinical adoption relies on both effective marketing and compelling research. Only 13.5% of consumers are considered early adopters—those willing to embrace innovation even before it has achieved product-market fit [6].

– Be patient. Great inventions take time. The manual typewriter (with the precedent QWERTY keyboard used to type this chapter) was patented in 1714, first commercialized in 1873, and not widely adopted until the late 1880s [4].

The culture of surgery is changing, with an increasing number of women entering the field, which will further reduce barriers for women in surgical innovation. Whether it's a leaky pipeline or a glass ceiling, we are all aware that there are too few women in leadership, academia, and, in this case, surgical innovation. Nevertheless, women continue to push boundaries and exhibit creativity.

Conclusion

While surgical innovation may not suit everyone, we hope this chapter has sparked your curiosity and encouraged you to explore a new and exciting path in your surgical career. Delving into research can ignite your curiosity, paving the way for groundbreaking solutions. Embracing surgical innovation calls for a hopeful outlook, empowering us to overcome challenges and build a brighter future for both our patients and ourselves. Let's inspire each other on this incredible journey!

References

1. 97% of Patents Never Make Money: How to Join the Elite 3%! (n.d.). Design 2 Market. Retrieved February 1, 2025, from https://www.design2market.co.uk/academy/97-of-patents-never-make-money/
2. Bell, A. M., Chetty, R., Jaravel, X., Petkova, N., & Van Reenen, J. (2017). *Who Becomes an Inventor in America? The Importance of Exposure to Innovation* (Working Paper 24062). National Bureau of Economic Research. https://doi.org/10.3386/w24062
3. Garcia-Ibáñez, R. (n.d.). Council Post: Five Essential Characteristics You'll Need To Bring An Invention To Market. Forbes. Retrieved February 1, 2025, from https://www.forbes.com/councils/forbesbusinesscouncil/2023/10/05/five-essential-characteristics-youll-need-to-bring-an-invention-to-market/
4. HNF – Typewriters – From the idea to a standard. (n.d.). Retrieved January 29, 2025, from https://www.hnf.de/en/permanent-exhibition/exhibition-areas/the-mechanization-of-information-technology/typewriters-from-the-idea-to-a-standard.html
5. Koning, R., Samila, S., & Ferguson, J.-P. (2021). Who do we invent for? Patents by women focus more on women's health, but few women get to invent. *Science (New York, N.Y.)*, *372*(6548), 1345–1348. https://doi.org/10.1126/science.aba6990
6. Rogers' Innovation Diffusion Theory (1962, 1995). (2024, November 21). ResearchGate. https://www.researchgate.net/publication/285171917_Rogers'_Innovation_Diffusion_Theory_1962_1995
7. Savage, R., & Wilson, A. (1977). Doctors' attitudes to women in medicine. *The Journal of the Royal College of General Practitioners*, *27*(179), 363–365.
8. Singh, C., Loseth, C., & Shoqirat, N. (2021). Women in surgery: A systematic review of 25 years. *BMJ Leader*, *5*(4), 283–290. https://doi.org/10.1136/leader-2019-000199

9. Soltani, T., Ratnasekera, A., Möller, M. G., Park, P. K., Russo, R. M., & Association of Women Surgeons Publications Committee. (2024). Women in surgical innovation: A guide to breaking down barriers and developing solutions from bench to bedside (Part I). *American Journal of Surgery*, 116012. https://doi.org/10.1016/j.amjsurg.2024.116012

10. Sugimoto, C. R., Ahn, Y.-Y., Smith, E., Macaluso, B., & Larivière, V. (2019). Factors affecting sex-related reporting in medical research: A cross-disciplinary bibliometric analysis. *The Lancet*, *393*(10171), 550–559. https://doi.org/10.1016/S0140-6736(18)32995-7

11. U.S. Physician Workforce Data Dashboard. (n.d.). AAMC. Retrieved January 29, 2025, from https://www.aamc.org/data-reports/report/us-physician-workforce-data-dashboard

12. Weinreich, H. M., Jin, V., Crowell, L., Skovlund, S. M., Williams, Q. L., & Buhimschi, I. A. (2023). Surgical Instrument Designers and Inventors—Where are the Women? *The American Surgeon™*, *89*(11), 4835–4841. https://doi.org/10.1177/00031348231172164

Chapter 21
Building Your Academic Career in Surgery Through Innovation and Scholarly Activity

Brianna R. Fram and Lisa K. Cannada

Introduction

> In the world of academic surgery, you're only as good as your last paper. —Anonymous

The pursuit of scholarly activity in surgery encompasses a broad spectrum of endeavors—from traditional original research to developing innovative educational materials for print and media, quality improvement initiatives, and surgical technique development. Summary publications, such as review papers and textbooks, and participation in debates by panel and invited commentary often follow an established record of scholarship in an area. It is important to realize that scholarly activity is not limited to those in academic medicine. These are pursuits and forms of lifelong learning that can be carried out in any practice setting.

For women in surgery, scholarly productivity represents both an opportunity and a challenge. While academic achievement creates pathways to leadership positions and professional recognition, disparities persist in publication rates, citation impact, and research funding between male and female surgeons [1–9].

This chapter explores how women surgeons can develop meaningful scholarly careers while navigating the unique barriers they face. Drawing from both evidence-based literature and personal experiences, it provides practical strategies for

B. R. Fram
Department of Orthopaedic Surgery and Rehabilitation Medicine, University of Chicago, Chicago, IL, USA
e-mail: brfram@gmail.com

L. K. Cannada (✉)
Department of Orthopaedics, University of North Carolina, Chapel Hill, NC, USA

Director of Faculty Integration, UNC SOM Charlotte, Charlotte, NC, USA

Novant Health Orthopaedic Fracture Clinic, Charlotte, NC, USA
e-mail: cannada.lisa@gmail.com

K. Yoon-Flannery et al. (eds.), *Women in Surgery*,
https://doi.org/10.1007/978-3-032-10971-2_21

establishing productive academic practices that align with career objectives and personal values. We will examine how the scholarly landscape is changing, with new metrics of impact and innovative platforms creating opportunities for women to contribute to surgical knowledge in ways that better accommodate diverse career paths.

The Value of Scholarly Activity in Surgical Careers

Scholarly activity serves multiple functions in a surgeon's career trajectory. Beyond the traditional view of research as a means to academic promotion, scholarly work allows surgeons to contribute to the field's advancement, establish professional identity, and develop networks that enhance clinical practice [10]. For women surgeons specifically, scholarly contributions offer an objective measure of expertise that can help overcome persistent gender biases in how surgical competence is perceived [11].

Participating in the academic conversation through publications, presentations, and educational innovation establishes one's presence in the field. As one female trauma surgeon reflected, "My research gave me a voice in spaces where I might otherwise be overlooked. Being introduced as 'the author of that paper on humerus fracture fixation' changed how colleagues interacted with me in the operating room." This connection between scholarly reputation and clinical respect illustrates why academic productivity is important for women building surgical careers.

The benefits extend beyond individual recognition. Women's participation in surgical scholarship has also expanded research priorities to include previously overlooked areas. Studies of sex differences in surgical outcomes, investigations into gender disparities in surgical training, and work-life integration have been welcomed as women's voices in academic surgery have increased. For example, sexual dysfunction following pelvic ring injuries has long been reported in men, but with minimal reporting in women. A groundbreaking series of papers by female orthopedic surgeons on outcomes after pelvic ring injuries in women identified high rates of dyspareunia and provided support for the safety of a trial vaginal delivery after these injuries [12, 13]. These contributions can not only enhance patient care across genders but also create more sustainable surgical career models for all practitioners.

Challenges for Women in Surgical Scholarship

Despite progress, women surgeons continue to face specific barriers to scholarly productivity. Understanding these challenges is the first step toward developing effective strategies to overcome them. These include time constraints, limited access to research networks, bias in the evaluation of work, and funding gaps. These challenges manifest in measurable disparities. In a review of the first and senior authors of the most cited studies in the top ten surgical journals from 2015 to 2020, there were 71.8% males as first authors and 82.3% males as senior authors [8]. A disturbing finding was that the gap between male first and senior authors widened over the time period. In a review specific to orthopedic surgery literature, from 2002 to 2021, analyzing 168,451 authors, there were 13.6% female first authors and 9.9% female senior authors [9]. What this article pointed out was noted papers with female first authors were more likely to have a female senior author. In contrast to the previous study, there was noted to be a significant positive trend in females as first authors.

Research Efficiency and Getting Over the Finish Line

When becoming involved in research, remember that while saying "yes" is important, it is essential to ensure project goals and expectations are clearly defined prior to beginning research. Saying yes to a research project or commencing a line of investigation without doing this can lead to aborted projects and unhappy collaborators. Protect your time, effort, and reputation by creating clarity before commencing a project. Key questions include (1) What are we asking? (2) What is the impact of the answer? (3) Is our proposed method of study adequate to answer this question? (4) How long do we anticipate adequate data collection will take? (5) How resource-intensive (in time, materials, money) will this be? (6) What are the planned figures or tables for a resulting publication? (7) What is the mode of dissemination of results? Target journals, meeting presentations, etc. (8) Who will be primarily responsible for each role (data collection, analysis, manuscript writing, submission, and response to reviewers), and (9) what is the intended order of authorship?

The following framework provides practical guidance for developing sustainable scholarly practices:

Define Your Scholarly Identity

Effective scholarly careers begin with intentional focus, rather than pursuing disconnected projects based on opportunity alone.

1. *Align scholarly work with clinical practice*: Select research questions that naturally emerge from your clinical work, creating synergy between patient care and academic productivity.
2. *Leverage your unique perspective*: Consider how your experiences as a surgeon, including your identity, such as being a woman, might illuminate unexplored questions or approaches in your field.

3. *Balance innovation with continuation*: Building on existing research topics to make it easier to demonstrate relevance and secure resources.
4. *Conduct research as programs, not projects*: Avoid single projects on a given topic. Design research questions on multiple facets of a subject to allow for efficient experimental design and data collection. This increases the chances of performing impactful research.

Cultivate Strategic Collaborations

No successful surgeon-scholar works in isolation. Strategic collaboration multiplies productivity while distributing workload:

1. *Develop multidisciplinary networks*: Use the connections and relationships you build to foster a strong team.
2. *Use your clinical insights as a selling point*: As a clinician, you bring clinically focused ideas that can focus investigation by basic science colleagues. Having a clinician involved and a discrete clinical applicability of projects can be beneficial for basic scientists in applying for grant funding.
3. *Establish trainee research pipelines*: Creating structured research opportunities for medical students and residents generates preliminary data and publication opportunities while supporting the next generation.
4. *Join multi-institutional collaboratives*: Participating in established research networks provides access to larger studies and shared resources. Participating in regional or national organizations can provide access to these collaboratives through networking.
5. *Master efficiency techniques*: Given the unique time constraints faced by women surgeons, efficiency in scholarly work becomes particularly crucial.

Conclusion

Scholarly activity remains an essential component of surgical careers, particularly for women seeking to build a reputation and advance within academic institutions and organizations. Through strategic planning, effective collaboration, and intentional career development, women can build satisfying scholarly careers that contribute meaningfully to surgical knowledge. The path forward requires both individual strategies and systemic changes. Women surgeons must advocate for themselves while institutions simultaneously work to eliminate structural barriers to scholarly productivity. By addressing both dimensions of this challenge, we can create an academic surgical environment where scholarly achievement reflects talent and dedication rather than gender.

References

1. Campbell RA, Helstrom E, Chew L, Eapen R, Plimack E, Correa A, Kutikov A, Abbosh P, Calaway A, Nizam A, Gupta S, Psutka SP, Barata P, Dizman N, Sindhani M, Weight CJ, Bukavina L. Gender Disparities in Citations and Altmetric Attention Score in Oncology. JCO Oncol Pract. 2025 Apr 10:OP2400767. https://doi.org/10.1200/OP-24-00767. Epub ahead of print. PMID: 40209147.
2. Santonocito C, Giambra MM, Lumia MG, Sanfilippo F, Fabbro VD, Rubulotta F, Bignami EG, Abelardo D, Lefrant JY, Rello J. Gender imbalance in critical care medicine journals. Anaesth Crit Care Pain Med. 2025 Mar 12:101504. https://doi.org/10.1016/j.accpm.2025.101504. Epub ahead of print. PMID: 40086731.
3. Kim G, Goodman E, Adams A, Skendelas J, Ward J, Wang F, Lu SE, In H. Gender Gap in Academic Surgery: Disparities in Early-Career Scholarly Productivity Sets the Stage for Unequal Academic Advancement. J Surg Res. 2024 Dec;304:356–364. https://doi.org/10.1016/j.jss.2024.10.035. Epub 2024 Nov 29. PMID: 39615152.
4. Freire CVS, Campos LN, Rangel AG, Naus A, Wagemaker S, Brandão GR, Schlindwein SS, Feres B, de Araújo Grisi G, Mooney DP, Ferreira JL, Ferreira R. Uncovering gaps in women's authorship: A big data analysis in academic surgery. World J Surg. 2024 Sep;48(9):2152–2162. https://doi.org/10.1002/wjs.12256. Epub 2024 Jun 23. PMID: 38923616.
5. Pickel L, Sivachandran N. Gender representation in Canadian surgical leadership and medical faculties: a cross-sectional study. BMC Med Educ. 2024 Jun 17;24(1):667. https://doi.org/10.1186/s12909-024-05641-6. PMID: 38886676; PMCID: PMC11184682.
6. Changez MIK, Toor AS, Tiwana M, Masud S, Wooding DJ, Khosa F. National institutes of health: Analysis of gender differences in anesthesiology research funding. Women Health. 2025 Feb;65(2):208–218. https://doi.org/10.1080/03630242.2025.2460664. Epub 2025 Feb 1. PMID: 39891539.
7. Oliveira DFM, Ma Y, Woodruff TK, Uzzi B. Comparison of National Institutes of Health Grant Amounts to First-Time Male and Female Principal Investigators. Number of publications female surgeons. JAMA. 2019 Mar 5;321(9):898–900. https://doi.org/10.1001/jama.2018.21944. PMID: 30835300; PMCID: PMC6439593.
8. Sauder M, Newsome K, Zagales I, Autrey C, Das S, Zagales R, Bilski T, Elkbuli A. Gender Distribution of First and Senior Authorship Across Most Cited Studies Within the Top Ten Surgical Journals From 2015–2020: Cementing Women Academic Surgery Representation. J Surg Res. 2022 Sep;277:7–16. https://doi.org/10.1016/j.jss.2022.03.019. Epub 2022 Apr 19.PMID: 35453056
9. Ghattas YS, Kyin C, Grise A, Glasser J, Johnson T, Druskovich K, Cannada LK, Service B. Trends in Female Authorship in Orthopaedic Literature from 2002 to 2021: An Analysis of 168,451 Authors. J Bone Joint Surg Am. 2023 Aug 16;105(16):1285–1294. https://doi.org/10.2106/JBJS.22.01290. Epub 2023 May 8.PMID: 37155604
10. McKenzie N, Dorsey C, Guerrero S, Donington J, Alverdy J, Nordgren R, Matthews JB, Baird BJ. Enhancing equity in academic surgery promotion practices. Surgery. 2025 Apr;180:109023. https://doi.org/10.1016/j.surg.2024.109023. Epub 2025 Jan 20. PMID: 39837048.
11. Madanay F, Bundorf MK, Ubel PA. Physician Gender and Patient Perceptions of Interpersonal and Technical Skills in Online Reviews. JAMA Netw Open. 2025 Feb 3;8(2):e2460018. https://doi.org/10.1001/jamanetworkopen.2024.60018. PMID: 39951262; PMCID: PMC11829228.
12. Vallier HA, Cureton BA, Schubeck D. Pelvic ring injury is associated with sexual dysfunction in women. J Orthop Trauma. 2012 May;26(5):308–13. https://doi.org/10.1097/BOT.0b013e31821d700e. PMID: 22011632.
13. Vallier HA, Cureton BA, Schubeck D. Pregnancy outcomes after pelvic ring injury. J Orthop Trauma. 2012 May;26(5):302–7. https://doi.org/10.1097/BOT.0b013e31822428c5. PMID: 22048182.

Chapter 22
Multicenter Clinical Trials

Jacklyn M. Engelbart and Pauline K. Park

Introduction

This chapter introduces multicenter clinical trials spanning conceptualization, design, and special consideration. Clinical trials are employed as a research method to answer well-defined, novel, ethical research questions that arise from findings of observational studies or early research work. Multicenter clinical trials in surgery may be used for the study of procedures, devices, care protocols, medications, and interventions. Multicenter clinical trials allow for more robust research with larger sample sizes, diverse populations, and result in more generalizable study outcomes. In addition to excellent study design, success is enhanced by a feasible design and strong implementation teams with collaborators and mentors who have the necessary expertise. Herein, we will explore the unique aspects of a multicenter clinical trial.

After defining a research question and the significance of the study, researchers embark on the study design. Studies are structured with specific selection criteria, sampling, duration, variables, and outcomes. In clinical trials, an intervention is selected and applied, and its effects and associations are studied. The approach for clinical trials varies by study question, with randomized, blinded clinical trial designs having the ability to provide the most definitive causal inference and minimizing confounding variable influence; however, some research questions may

J. M. Engelbart
Department of Surgery, University of Iowa, Iowa City, IA, USA
e-mail: engelbar@med.umich.edu

P. K. Park (✉)
Professor of Surgery, Co-Director Surgical Intensive Care Unit, Program Director, Surgical Critical Care Fellowship, Department of Surgery, Division of Acute Care Surgery, University of Michigan, Ann Arbor, MI, USA
e-mail: parkpk@med.umich.edu

K. Yoon-Flannery et al. (eds.), *Women in Surgery*,
https://doi.org/10.1007/978-3-032-10971-2_22

necessitate nonrandomized or unblinded studies for feasibility. Alternative study designs, including within-group studies, cross-over studies, pilot studies, and non-randomized between-group study designs. Study outcomes with strong internal validity and generalizability can be attributed to well-crafted multicenter clinical trial study designs. The results from these studies form a basis for future practice guidelines.

Multicenter clinical trial design requires carefully coordinated efforts for the selection of participating centers, randomization, centralized or decentralized data collection, and protocol adherence across participating centers. Pilot studies provide an opportunity to determine the feasibility of a trial and the acceptability of the interventions. Participating center selection in multicenter clinical trials in surgery involves not only considering the patient population but also the services that can be provided at the center and the feasibility of recruitment and protocol adherence. Randomization can be done off-site to minimize bias. Blinding can be difficult with clinical trials in surgery, especially in studies assessing procedural interventions or devices. Data collection has evolved over time with considerations of centralized or decentralized data collection and a more recent focus on managing big data in clinical trials, as well as the incorporation of data from real-time monitoring. Centralized databases can be used to manage study data, and data monitoring committees are essential in multicenter clinical trials in surgery. Interim monitoring by this committee helps to ensure study quality, consistency across participating centers, and protocol adherence and can determine if it is necessary to stop a trial early. Statistical analyses can be done via intention-to-treat and per-protocol analyses, as well as subgroup analyses, which can help discover effect modification.

While strong study designs, collaboration, and a successful intervention can lead to completion of a practice-changing clinical trial, challenges exist in conducting multicenter surgical trials. Recruitment of study participants presents challenges, such as sample size requirements, participants with a lack of decision-making capacity, or extreme variability in the populations at participating sites. Patient consent processes and ethical review boards must be coordinated among participating sites. Challenges exist with implementation, including measurement variation and difficulties with protocol adherence. When coordinating multicenter clinical trials in surgery, differences may exist in institutional capabilities and resources, which can affect implementation. In multicenter clinical trials, a coordinating center establishes the operational details of the study and the communication, trains the staff, ensures quality control, and oversees data collection, management, and analysis. Steering committees and subcommittees can also help to coordinate and address challenges, especially those related to study quality control and training, as well as manage publications, presentations, and additional studies with secondary data analysis.

Is there a role for collaboration between surgeons, researchers, and industry? Absolutely, there is also a role for the Food and Drug Administration (FDA) and other regulatory bodies in surgical trials. Multicenter clinical trials in surgery are done to test the effectiveness and safety of new treatments and, in consideration of approval by regulatory bodies, are subject to regulatory requirements. The FDA and regulatory bodies provide guidelines for this research. There are multiple stages in investigating new therapeutic interventions. The preclinical phase studies an intervention in tissues and animals. Phase I studies include testing in a small group of volunteers for safety. Phase II studies include a small study to test intervention tolerability and dosage. Phase III studies include large randomized clinical trials to demonstrate that the benefits outweigh the risks of the intervention. Phase III trials are used as a basis for FDA approval. Phase IV clinical trials are observational studies to confirm the benefits and study rare adverse effects of the intervention.

Special Considerations for Multicenter Surgical Clinical Trials

Recruitment and follow-up in multicenter clinical trials in surgery can take many forms. In some trials, patients are not able to provide informed consent, and community consent is needed. In some trials, patients may be more likely to be lost to follow-up, and thus, careful planning to retain patients within the trial can reduce some of these limitations. Blinding and randomization can be particularly challenging in multicenter surgical clinical trials, but in some trials, randomization can occur prior to surgeons seeing patients. Blinding can sometimes occur with the patient, the physician assessor, or the outcome assessor.

As with all research, ethical research is imperative. The ethical principles published in the Belmont Report, including respect for persons, beneficence, and justice, have provided the foundation for ethical research conduct [1]. In the case of consent, these principles are followed by providing possible research participants with all relevant information for the study needed to fully comprehend and be able to make a voluntary decision about whether to participate in the study. Risks and benefits of the research must be disclosed during the consent process. The selection of subjects should be as equitable as possible. Conflicts of interest should be avoided and appropriate disclosures made as necessary.

Study timelines should take into consideration the timeframe needed for protocol preparation, training, recruitment, clinical interventions, data analysis, and dissemination of the results through publication, presentations, and other forms of communication of study results (Fig. 22.1). While it is impossible to deliver the same surgery or procedural intervention to every patient enrolled in a clinical trial, it is helpful to establish operational definitions and standardize diagnostic testing, medical treatment, and surgical treatment across all centers included in surgical critical trials. Considerations may be given to control for surgeons' experience or to assess the quality of the intervention performed. Failure to assess and control the delivery and quality of the intervention may significantly affect outcomes.

Multicenter clinical trials in surgery provide a research method through which a team of physicians, researchers, industry, and government or regulatory agencies, as collaborators, can evaluate an intervention's safety and efficacy across multiple centers with the same study protocol. These studies require a large number of resources, collaboration, and expertise. Carefully constructed multicenter clinical trials in

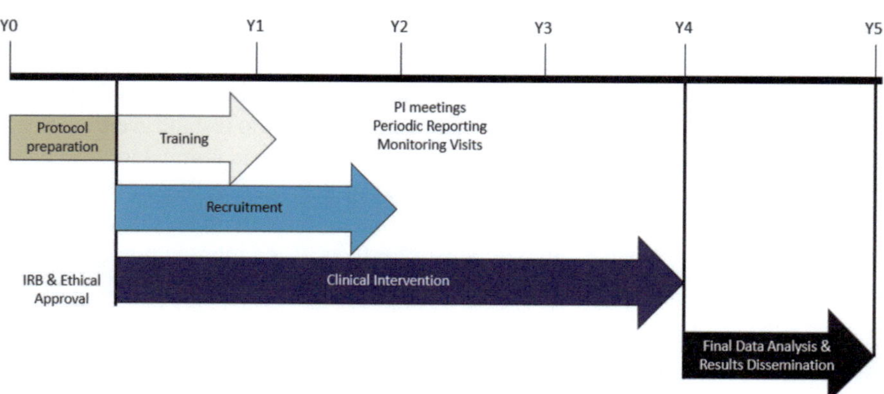

Fig. 22.1 Sample study timeline

surgery take into consideration data management complexity and ethical considerations, especially with informed consent, and attempt to mitigate site variability with regard to study protocols, treatment practices, and surgical techniques. The resulting outcomes are more generalizable and comprehensive when compared to single-center studies and can inform changes in evidence-based practice guidelines.

Reference

1. The National Commission for the Protection of Human Subjects of Biomedical and Behavioral Research. (1979) The Belmont Report: Ethical Principles and Guidelines for the Protection of Human Subjects of Research. https://www.hhs.gov/ohrp/regulations-and-policy/belmont-report/read-the-belmont-report/index.html

Part VI

Global Perspectives on Women in Surgery

Chapter 23
Cultural and Societal Factors Impacting Women in Surgery Worldwide

Neelam Mulji and Lucy M. De La Cruz

Introduction

Despite the undeniable progress toward gender equity in medicine, surgery remains a traditionally male-dominated specialty. Globally, women constitute approximately 30% of surgical trainees [7], yet often encounter systemic, cultural, and societal barriers that impede their career advancement. These disparities are not only rooted in individual choices but also deeply embedded in cultural norms, stereotypes, and institutional structures. Surgery's historically perceived physical demands, hierarchical culture, and associated traits of decisiveness and endurance have further perpetuated gendered perceptions aligning the field with masculinity [11].

This chapter explores the impact of culture and society on women in surgery worldwide, highlighting both shared challenges and region-specific issues. By examining the intersections of gender, work-life balance, mentorship, patient perception, and systemic inequities, it aims to provide a global perspective on how women navigate—and reshape—the surgical profession.

N. Mulji
Breast Surgical Oncology Fellow, MedStar Georgetown University Hospital, Washington, DC, USA
e-mail: Neelam.j.Mulji@medstar.net

L. M. De La Cruz (✉)
Chief of Breast Surgery, MedStar Georgetown University Hospital, Washington, DC, USA

Associate Professor of Surgery, Georgetown University School of Medicine, Washington, DC, USA
e-mail: lucydlcb@gmail.com

K. Yoon-Flannery et al. (eds.), *Women in Surgery*,
https://doi.org/10.1007/978-3-032-10971-2_23

Gender Stereotypes and Professional Identity

The stereotype of the "surgical personality"—characterized by traits of decisiveness, physical stamina, and authoritative communication—has historically been associated with masculinity [1]. Such traits are stereotypically aligned with societal expectations of men, which influence both external perceptions of surgeons and the internalization of professional identity amongst women.

In Western countries, women surgeons are often subtly questioned about their competence or commitment. Evolving gender narratives have allowed female surgeons to challenge stereotypes, often serving as role models [10]. Conversely, in countries with rigid patriarchal norms—such as areas in the Middle East and South Asia—traditional gender roles persist, discouraging women from engaging fully in surgical specialties [6]. These cultural norms often extend into curricula, training environments, and patient perceptions, further entrenching stereotypes.

Breaking down gender stereotypes requires multifaceted approaches, including early exposure to surgical careers in medical education, mentorship programs, and media representation that portrays women as competent surgeons. Increasing evidence-based awareness can gradually shift societal perceptions [4].

Work-Life Balance and Family Expectations

Globally, women bear disproportionate responsibilities for motherhood and family and household management, often intersecting with their professional roles [9]. Research indicates that female surgeons frequently delay or limit clinical roles due to family commitments [11].

In Latin America, cultural emphasis on traditional gender roles can intensify scrutiny of female surgeons who "neglect" domestic duties. In Africa, where healthcare systems are already under-resourced, women face the dual pressures of community caregiving roles and clinical demands. Even in high-income countries, institutional support for work-life integration is inconsistent, and stigma around maternity leave persists.

Conversely, Scandinavian countries with more progressive family policies have seen higher retention of women in surgical specialties [12]. Institutional reforms such as flexible training schedules, subsidized child care, and parental leave policies have proven effective. Promoting a culture that values work-life balance, such as in Scandinavian countries, could prove fruitful to surgical departments worldwide.

Mentorship, Representation, and Leadership

Mentorship and visibility of female role models are crucial for breaking cycles of underrepresentation. In regions where women's participation in surgery is nascent, mentorship opportunities are scarce, further perpetuating gender disparities [8].

Women surgeons benefit immensely from mentors who can provide guidance, advocate for opportunities, and serve as role models demonstrating that leadership is attainable regardless of gender [2]. Organizations such as the Association of Women Surgeons (AWS), Women in Surgery Africa, and regional mentorship networks in Asia are creating opportunities for women to thrive.

Leadership roles, such as heads of departments, academic chairs, or society presidents, tend to be overwhelmingly occupied by men. An analysis by Butt et al. [3] revealed that globally, female surgical leaders constitute less than 20% of senior positions, despite comparable entry rates into training programs. Cultural factors—such as societal expectations and institutional biases—limit opportunities for women to ascend into top roles [10].

Structured mentorship programs, sponsorship initiatives, and intentional gender-balanced selection committees can promote leadership parity. Encouraging male allies to advocate for women and establishing leadership development programs aimed at women can effectively challenge systemic biases.

Patient Perceptions and Cultural Acceptance

Cultural attitudes toward female physicians also affect patient trust and acceptance. In conservative societies, patients may prefer female surgeons for gender-concordant care but resist their authority in high-stakes specialties such as cardiac or trauma surgery. Consequently, patients are more accepting of female surgeons in roles like breast surgery, based on comfort and communication [10]. Even in Western contexts with higher gender equality norms, patients may unconsciously assume a woman surgeon is a nurse or trainee, reflecting persistent gender bias. To improve cultural acceptance, surgeons must develop culturally sensitive communication skills and provide evidence of competence through transparent interactions and patient education campaigns. Public awareness initiatives highlighting women's achievements in surgery can challenge stereotypes and enhance patient trust [4].

Structural and Institutional Barriers

Women in surgery encounter systemic inequities ranging from unequal pay and promotion opportunities to a lack of maternity leave policies. In low- and middle-income countries, these inequities are compounded by limited infrastructure, unsafe workplaces, and fewer academic pathways, which disproportionately hinder women's advancement. These restrictions hinder the participation of women in surgical specialization.

Embedding gender equity into institutional missions, providing childcare facilities, and ensuring equitable pay are proven strategies that improve retention and advancement of women in surgery [4, 5].

Conclusion

The representation of women in surgery is not simply a workforce issue—it reflects the broader cultural and societal forces shaping women's roles in professional and public life.

Recognizing and addressing these challenges requires both structural reforms and cultural change.

Resilience amongst women surgeons—further fielded by international organizations, mentorship networks, and advocacy—continues to drive change. Creating culturally sensitive and inclusive environments enables female surgeons worldwide to thrive, eventually transforming the surgical landscape into one characterized by true gender parity.

References

1. Bar-On, S., Lev, S., & Hazan, H. (2007). The surgical personality: Myth or reality? *Journal of Surgical Education, 64*(5), 356–362. https://doi.org/10.1016/j.jsurg.2007.05.006
2. Buchanan, C. D., Stallworth, J. L., Christophel, J. J., Dacus, J. W., & Jackson, R. S. (2018). Mentorship in surgery: A survey of mentors and mentees. *American Journal of Surgery, 215*(1), 140–144. https://doi.org/10.1016/j.amjsurg.2017.05.015
3. Butt, Z., Ashraf, H., Khan, A., & Malik, A. A. (2020). Gender disparity in surgical leadership worldwide: Where do we stand? *World Journal of Surgery, 44*(11), 3620–3628. https://doi.org/10.1007/s00268-020-05695-3
4. Gaynor, M., Seabury, S. A., & Jena, A. B. (2017). The gender gap in surgical careers: Evidence, implications, and interventions. *JAMA Surgery, 152*(12), 1086–1087. https://doi.org/10.1001/jamasurg.2017.3900
5. Goyal, R., Mateen, F. J., & Rai, A. (2021). Barriers to advancement of women in surgery: A global perspective. *The Lancet Global Health, 9*(5), e634–e635. https://doi.org/10.1016/S2214-109X(21)00097-2
6. Khan, F., Qureshi, H., & Rehman, A. (2021). Gender roles and women in surgical training in South Asia. *BMJ Global Health, 6*(4), e004329. https://doi.org/10.1136/bmjgh-2020-004329
7. Mowatt, G., Bunker, J., & Fish, R. (2002). Women in surgical training: An international perspective. *World Journal of Surgery, 26*(2), 151–155. https://doi.org/10.1007/s00268-001-0195-3
8. Nguyen, T. C., McKenney, J. M., & Williams, J. R. (2019). The role of mentorship for women in surgical training: A global review. *Annals of Surgery, 270*(1), 102–108. https://doi.org/10.1097/SLA.0000000000003262
9. Ofori-Amoah, V., Boateng, R., & Nortey, P. (2018). Work–life balance challenges of women surgeons: A global exploration. *International Journal of Surgery, 52*, 35–39. https://doi.org/10.1016/j.ijsu.2018.01.017
10. Princip, M., & Turney, B. (2012). Gender stereotypes in surgical training: Cultural perspectives. *Medical Education, 46*(12), 1185–1193. https://doi.org/10.1111/medu.12023
11. Vaidya, J. S., Lakhani, S. R., & Holmberg, L. (2017). Women in surgery: Overcoming barriers. *The Lancet, 389*(10087), 774–776. https://doi.org/10.1016/S0140-6736(17)30608-1
12. Auchus, R., Karlsson, M., & Lindgren, A. (2019). Family policies and female surgeon retention: Lessons from Scandinavia. *Scandinavian Journal of Surgery, 108*(3), 189–196. https://doi.org/10.1177/1457496918821247

13. Sullivan, G. M., & Artino, A. R., Jr. (2017). Gender differences in academic surgery, work-life balance, division of household duties, and satisfaction. *Journal of Surgical Research, 218,* 99–107. https://doi.org/10.1016/j.jss.2017.07.041
14. Oppenheimer-Velez, M., Sims, C., Labiner, H., Baxter, N., Kozar, R., McCoy, J., Sanfey, H., Litle, V., Klingensmith, M., & Pories, S. (2022). Women empowering women: Assessing the American College of Surgeons Women in Surgery Committee Mentorship Program. *Journal of the American College of Surgeons, 235*(2), 375–381. https://doi.org/10.1097/XCS.0000000000000272
15. Case, M., Herrera, M., Rumps, M. V., & Mulcahey, M. K. (2024). The Impact of Mentoring on Academic Career Success in Surgical Subspecialties: A Systematic Review. *Journal of surgical education, 81*(12), 103292. https://doi.org/10.1016/j.jsurg.2024.09.011

Chapter 24
Access to Surgical Education and Training in Different Regions

Sylvia A. Reyes

The United States has long been recognized as a host to some of the best surgical training programs in the world; however, surgical education and training programs throughout this country are not equally dispersed. Significant disparities exist in surgical training programs by geography, gender, mentorship, and race/ethnicity, which eventually affect access, attrition rates, training quality, and career progression [1–6]. The lack of access to surgical education in certain areas of the USA contributes to the formation of medical deserts where access to care and the surgical workforce is limited [7–9]. In this chapter, we will learn more about these differences and what efforts are being made to address them.

Regional Distribution of Residency Programs

General surgical residency programs have historically been concentrated in urban and metropolitan areas where large teaching hospitals and academic medical centers are located, thus limiting the availability of surgical training in rural areas. More residency opportunities exist in regions with a high density of medical schools and hospitals, such as the Northeast (Boston, New York, Philadelphia), Midwest (Chicago, Cleveland), West Coast (San Francisco, Los Angeles), and South (Houston, Miami), as seen in Fig. 24.1 below from FREIDA™, the American Medical Association Residency and Fellowship Database.

This uneven distribution of residency programs in the United States has contributed to the widening gap in surgeon supply between rural and urban areas. An

S. A. Reyes (✉)

Director of Breast Services Health Equity Programs at Northwell Zuckerberg Cancer Center,
Assistant Professor of Surgery, Zucker School of Medicine at Hofstra, Long Island, NY, USA
e-mail: sylviareyesmd@gmail.com

K. Yoon-Flannery et al. (eds.), *Women in Surgery*,
https://doi.org/10.1007/978-3-032-10971-2_24

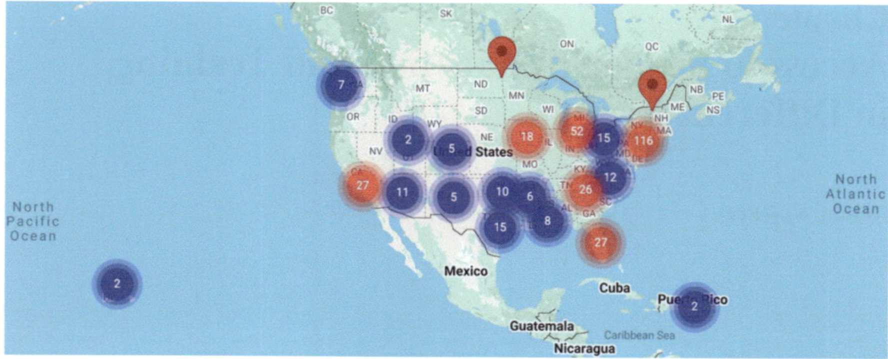

Fig. 24.1 Regional distribution of surgical residency programs in the United States. (https://freida.ama-assn.org/search/map?spec=43326&loc=01,02,03,04,05,06,07,08,09,PR&markersLoaded =true&mapMarkerCount=368)

analysis of the National Resident Matching Program and Association of American Medical Colleges databases from 2012 to 2019 found that General Surgery experienced a slower growth of residents and simultaneous decreases in practicing physicians and workforce overall, suggesting that the current population growth rate is exceeding the rate of physicians entering GS and particularly hurting rural areas [8]. Similarly, a population-based study of all US counties from 2010 to 2020 found that the number of surgeons per capita has decreased in rural counties and increased in urban counties over time, thereby exacerbating access issues in underserved regions [7]. This increase in county-level social vulnerability has been associated with worse surgical outcomes, especially among minority patients [10].

Disparities in Gender and Race: Attrition and Operative Experience

Not only are there differences in the geographic distribution of residency programs, but there are also significant disparities in who is admitted into these programs and who ultimately completes them. According to the AAMC, women make up nearly a quarter (22.6%) of active general surgeons. However, higher attrition rates among female surgical trainees compared to their male counterparts suggest that the number of women in surgery could have been greater. A comprehensive study analyzing 18 years of data (2001–2018) from the AAMC found that the proportion of female surgical residents increased to a mean of 40% over time [6]. Overall attrition rate among all specialties was 6.9%, with an unintended attrition rate (withdrawals or dismissals unrelated to career change) of 2.3%. Female residents were at significantly higher risk of both overall attrition (RR 1.16) and unintended attrition (RR 1.17).

Residents who were underrepresented in medicine (URiM) comprised 14.9% (16,695) of all surgical trainees but demonstrated a 2.1% decrease over the study period. URiM residents had an even higher risk: overall attrition (RR 1.40) and unintended attrition (RR 1.92). Black/African American residents were particularly vulnerable, with unintended attrition risks over 2.5 times higher than their peers (RR 2.59). These findings underscore the urgent need for targeted strategies to recruit, retain, and support women and URiM trainees.

Further disparities are evident in operative experience. A multi-institutional analysis of the Accreditation Council for Graduate Medical Education case logs of 1343 categorical general surgery residents from 2010 to 2020, compared total/surgeon-chief/surgeon-junior case volumes between racial/ethnic groups [4]. Among the resident cohort, there were 211 (15.7%) Asian, 65 (4.8%) Black, 73 (5.4%) Hispanic, 71 (5.3%) "Other" (Native American or Multiple Race), and 923 (68.7%) White residents. Black residents were found to have significantly lower operative experience with 76 fewer total cases and 69 fewer surgeon junior cases ($P < 0.001$) than White residents. Although operative volume increased across all groups over time, the gap between racial groups persisted. These discrepancies in training may hinder future job opportunities and board passage rates. Organizations such as The National Council for Residents have formed specialty councils and teams of advisors to address these gaps by supporting residents in danger of attrition, but broader systemic changes are necessary to ensure equitable training experiences.

Mentorship Gaps and Their Implications

Effective mentorship is critical to surgical training, yet disparities in access to mentorship continue to affect trainee well-being and success. A 2019 survey of over 6000 general surgery residents revealed that one-third lacked meaningful mentorship [5]. This deficit was especially pronounced among non-White and Hispanic trainees. The presence of meaningful mentorship significantly correlated with increased perceptions of operative autonomy (OR 3.87) and reduced odds of burnout (OR 0.52), thoughts of attrition (OR 0.42), and suicidality (OR 0.47). These data emphasize the vital role mentorship plays in resident development and retention and point to an area ripe for intervention.

Regional Differences in Surgical Workforce and Compensation

The imbalance in the distribution of the surgical workforce is also influenced by regional differences in compensation, working conditions, and professional support. Lower compensation and fewer professional development opportunities in rural and underserved areas discourage surgeon recruitment and retention. This dynamic exacerbates already strained healthcare systems in these regions and contributes to persistent health inequities [8].

Future research is needed to better assess the relationship between workforce distribution, patient outcomes, and the impact of recent policies aimed at alleviating provider shortages. Continued monitoring and policy innovation will be crucial to bridging this gap.

Initiatives to Address Regional Disparities

Several promising efforts are underway to address persistent geographic and demographic disparities in surgical education and workforce distribution. These initiatives span from structural innovations in training pathways to leveraging technological tools, all aiming to improve access to surgical care in underserved communities.

One key strategy involves expanding residency programs in Medically Underserved Areas (MUAs). The Accreditation Council for Graduate Medical Education (ACGME) has implemented initiatives to support training in these regions, encouraging the development of residency programs where the physician workforce is most needed. In 2019, the ACGME approved a framework to support the development of GME programs that enhance access to care in MUAs [12, 13].

Another important effort is the creation of rural surgical training pathways. Dedicated rural tracks and rural rotations are increasingly incorporated into general surgery residencies to prepare physicians for practice in rural settings [8]. A national survey of General Surgery Program Directors found that about 28% of the 41% of ACGME-accredited surgery programs that responded to the survey offer some rural exposure—ranging from dedicated tracks to required or elective rural rotations—with variability in structure and duration [14]. Specialized programs, such as the North Dakota rural track, demonstrated high trainee satisfaction: among surveyed graduates, 83% entered the rural track with a desire to practice rurally, and 75% ultimately practiced in rural communities [15]. Additional systematic reviews show that rural surgical rotations during residency are associated with a more than two-fold increase in surgeons practicing in rural areas (odds ratio 2.19) [16–18].

Integrating education on health disparities and community health into medical curricula has emerged as another lever for change. A cross-sectional study of over 48,000 graduating medical students interested in surgery found that women and students from underrepresented racial and ethnic groups—or those with global health or disparities experiences—were more likely to express intentions to practice in underserved areas. These findings underscore the importance of medical schools and residency programs embracing their social and clinical missions to diversify the surgical workforce and improve access to care [11, 19].

Technological innovation is also transforming surgical training. Virtual reality (VR) and artificial intelligence (AI) tools are increasingly used to enhance skills training. For example, a landmark study by Seymour et al. [20] demonstrated that VR simulation significantly improved the performance of novice laparoscopists in a controlled environment. Similarly, the Touch Surgery™ app was validated for cognitive training in laparoscopic procedures, offering a scalable and accessible learning tool [21]. Additionally, a rapid review showed that online modules teaching surgical skills to clinical-year medical students can supplement or partially compensate for limited hands-on training, especially in constrained settings [22].

Conclusion

Access to surgical education in the United States is shaped by geographic, racial, and gender-based disparities that limit equitable training and workforce distribution. These structural barriers compromise not only the development of future surgeons but also the quality of surgical care in underserved regions. Addressing these challenges requires a multifaceted approach that includes expanding residency opportunities in MUAs, investing in mentorship and support systems, advancing equity in operative experience, and leveraging technology to equalize access to quality surgical training. A concerted national effort to recruit, train, and retain a diverse surgical workforce—especially in rural and underserved regions—is essential for building a more inclusive and effective surgical healthcare system.

References

1. Elkbuli A, Rhodes H, Breeding T, Ngatuvai M, Beeton G, Rosander A, Maka P, Alter N, Havron W. Analysis of Racial and Gender Distribution of US MD Graduates Entering Into General Surgery and Surgical Subspecialties Residencies: The Need for Effective & Sustainable Diversity, Equity, and Inclusion Strategies. J Surg Res. 2023 Sep;289:141–151. doi: https://doi.org/10.1016/j.jss.2023.03.044. Epub 2023 Apr 27. PMID: 37119615.
2. Saif A, Sarvestani AL, Teke ME, Copeland AR, Gupta S, Shindorf ML, Eade AV, Juneau P, Jean-Jacques A, Blakely AM, Hernandez JM. Sex and Race/Ethnicity Based Trends in Matriculation to General Surgery Residency and Associated Fellowship Programs. J Surg Res. 2024 Dec;304:297–304. doi: https://doi.org/10.1016/j.jss.2024.10.020. Epub 2024 Nov 22. PMID: 39579469.
3. Zmijewski P, Park YS, Hogan S, Holmboe E, Klingensmith M, Cortez A, Lindeman B, Chen H, Smith B, Fazendin J. Trends in Operative Case Logs of Chief Residents in Surgery by Sex and Race: A 5-year National Study. Ann Surg. 2024 Sep 1;280(3):473–479. doi: https://doi.org/10.1097/SLA.0000000000006373. Epub 2024 Jul 3. PMID: 38957982.
4. Eruchalu CN, Etheridge JC, Hammaker AC, Kader S, Abelson JS, Harvey J, Farr D, Stopenski SJ, Nahmias JT, Elsaadi A, Campbell SJ, Foote DC, Ivascu FA, Montgomery KB, Zmijewski P, Byrd SE, Kimbrough MK, Smith S, Postlewait LM, Dodwad SM, Adams SD, Markesbery KC, Meister KM, Woeste MR, Martin RCG 2nd, Callahan ZM, Marks JA, Patel P, Anstadt MJ, Nasim BW, Willis RE, Patel JA, Newcomb MR, Stahl CC, Yafi MA, Sutton JM, George BC, Quillin RC 3rd, Cho NL, Cortez AR. Racial and Ethnic Disparities in Operative Experience Among General Surgery Residents: A Multi-Institutional Study from the US ROPE Consortium.

Ann Surg. 2024 Jan 1;279(1):172–179. doi: https://doi.org/10.1097/SLA.0000000000005848. Epub 2023 Mar 17. PMID: 36928294; PMCID: PMC11104265.

5. Silver CM, Yuce TK, Clarke CN, et al. Disparities in Mentorship and Implications for US Surgical Resident Education and Wellness. JAMA Surg. 2024;159(6):687–695. doi:https://doi.org/10.1001/jamasurg.2024.0533

6. Haruno LS, Chen X, Metzger M, et al. Racial and Sex Disparities in Resident Attrition Among Surgical Subspecialties. JAMA Surg. 2023;158(4):368–376. doi:https://doi.org/10.1001/jamasurg.2022.7640

7. Patel VR, Liu M, Byrne JP, Haynes AB, Ibrahim AM. Surgeon Supply by County-Level Rurality and Social Vulnerability From 2010 to 2020. JAMA Surg. 2024;159(2):223–225. doi:https://doi.org/10.1001/jamasurg.2023.5632

8. Zagales I, Bourne M, Sutherland M, et al. Regional Population-Based Workforce Shortages in General Surgery by Practicing Surgeon and Resident Trainee. The American SurgeonTM. 2021;87(6):855–863. doi:https://doi.org/10.1177/00031348211029870

9. Johnson SM, Miller-Hammond K. The State of Surgical Care Access in America: Current Challenges, Disparities, and Emerging Solutions. The American Surgeon. 2025;91(6):925–927. doi:https://doi.org/10.1177/00031348251331283

10. Diaz A, Hyer JM, Barmash E, Azap R, Paredes AZ, Pawlik TM. County-level social vulnerability is associated with worse surgical outcomes, especially among minority patients. Ann Surg. 2021;274(6):881–891. doi:https://doi.org/10.1097/SLA.0000000000004691

11. Nguyen M, Cerasani M, Dinka LA, et al. Association of Demographic Factors and Medical School Experiences With Students' Intention to Pursue a Surgical Specialty and Practice in Underserved Areas. JAMA Surg. 2021;156(12):e214898. doi:https://doi.org/10.1001/jamasurg.2021.4898

12. ACGME. Medically Underserved Areas initiatives targeting residency distribution in underserved regions: https://www.acgme.org/initiatives/medically-underserved-areas-and-populations/

13. Abid, M., Rodefeld, L., Adhikari, M., Jarman, B., McDougal, L., O'Rourke, A. P., Amiri, F., & Hawes, E. M. (2025). Cultivating Rural Surgeons: An Analysis of the Current Rural Surgery Graduate Medical Education Landscape and a Roadmap to Program Creation. Journal of surgical education, 82(4), 103446. https://doi.org/10.1016/j.jsurg.2025.103446

14. Heller, S. F., Brasel, K. J., Dissanaike, S., & Fox, C. A. (2025). Rural Surgery Experiences in General Surgery Residency Training-The Current State an ACGME Sponsored Survey of General Surgery Program Directors. Journal of surgical education, 82(3), 103392. https://doi.org/10.1016/j.jsurg.2024.103392

15. Clark, N. M., McClure, P., Erickson, A., Andrilla, H. A., Riha, G., Dennis, A., Stewart, B. T., Lynge, D. C., & Patterson, D. G. (2025). Impact of Rural Exposure During General Surgery Residency on Practice in a Rural Community. Annals of surgery, 282(2), 186–192. https://doi.org/10.1097/SLA.0000000000006696

16. Resnick AS, Corrigan D, He J, et al. A survey of rural training opportunities in general surgery residency programs. J Surg Educ. 2024;81(2):297–305. doi:https://doi.org/10.1016/j.jsurg.2023.10.002

17. Barber JC, Velez DR, Johnson SW, et al. Effectiveness of a dedicated rural general surgery residency track: a 13-year analysis in North Dakota. Am Surg. 2025;91(2):122–129. doi:https://doi.org/10.1177/00031348231234567

18. George BC, Bohnen JD, Williams RG, et al. Rural surgical rotations during residency and odds of rural practice: a systematic review and meta-analysis. JAMA Surg. 2023;158(2):e225492. doi:https://doi.org/10.1001/jamasurg.2022.5492

19. Xierali IM, Nivet MA. Using diversity-related experiences to predict practice intentions of medical graduates. JAMA Surg. 2018;153(4):300–305. doi:https://doi.org/10.1001/jamasurg.2017.5040

20. Seymour NE, Gallagher AG, Roman SA, et al. Virtual reality training improves operating room performance: results of a randomized, double-blinded study. Ann Surg. 2002;236(4):458–464. doi:https://doi.org/10.1097/00000658-200210000-00008
21. Kowalewski KF, Hendrie JD, Schmidt MW, et al. Validation of the mobile serious game application Touch Surgery™ for cognitive training and assessment of laparoscopic cholecystectomy. Surg Endosc. 2017;31(11):4526–4532. doi:https://doi.org/10.1007/s00464-017-5548-3
22. Co M, Kwok K, Cheng B. Online learning for surgical skill in clinical-year medical students: a rapid review. Med Sci Educ. 2024;34(1):1–9. doi:https://doi.org/10.1007/s40670-024-01789-x

Part VII
Advocacy and Leadership in Surgery

Chapter 25
Promotion

Kahyun Yoon-Flannery

Promotion is a part of our academic medicine career. From an Instructor of Surgery, who is usually provided at the level of a junior attending or a fellow attending still in training, all the way to a full Professor of Surgery, there are usually strict guidelines that are provided by each institution.

Faculty Affairs offices in each institution usually will have the means to facilitate any initial faculty appointments and discuss any requirements for the promotion process. Many institutions will provide an annual workshop focusing on specific requirements for promotion.

There are usually three main tracks for promotion in Academic Surgery. First is the Clinical/Educator track, where the requirements usually involve clinical excellence with some teaching involved. Second, the research track usually involves a track for surgeon scientists who have funded research and publications. Lastly, there is a clinician track, where the focus remains mostly on clinical work and service to the institution in general. Clinical track may still involve a full-time clinical faculty; however, there is less pressure and focus on high-volume research.

As you are starting your career, it is incredibly helpful to identify a mentor in your field, if possible. Preferably, this mentor would be at least a level above your current rank and would be able to guide you in your planning for promotion and career planning in general. Early career faculty can provide excitement and energy to the department, but that energy can also be easily lost in the way if not harnessed properly.

Typically, in order to become an Assistant Professor of Surgery, you have to become board-certified and have 1–3 years of rank. For the Associate level, the expected time in rank is 5–7 years. For a full Professor, the typical time in rank is

K. Yoon-Flannery (✉)
Chief of Women's Cancer Services, Chief of Breast Surgery, Atlanticare Regional Medical Center, Egg Harbor Township, NJ, USA
e-mail: kay.yoonflannery@gmail.com

K. Yoon-Flannery et al. (eds.), *Women in Surgery*,
https://doi.org/10.1007/978-3-032-10971-2_25

10+ years. In addition to board certification, evidence of scholarly activity is critical, including peer-reviewed publications and participation in research, as well as excellence in teaching, which will be demonstrated in the teaching portfolio. It is incredibly valuable to start your teaching portfolio as soon as you start your career and start updating your curriculum vitae using a standard format. As you continue to increase your research and academic portfolio, remember to update your CV and portfolio with presentations, publications, and evaluations from your mentees as you complete them. It can be incredibly challenging to track down your previous commitments at the time of application.

It is also customary to require applicants to provide at least three colleagues who can serve as references. It should be noted that in most cases, someone outside of your institution will be required to provide a letter for you. It is not uncommon to see surgeons struggling to find someone outside of their own institution to write a recommendation letter. This should provide an incentive to continue networking in your area of expertise on both the regional and national levels.

A summary statement is also customarily required as a part of the promotion application package. This typically should be a summary outlining your accomplishments, particularly showing highlights of your career. A teaching dossier is also something that can be a requirement, including examples of any presentations or lectures you may have provided.

Promotion is a critical milestone in an academic surgical career. Staying organized and intentional in your approach to advancement is essential to navigating this process. It is important not only to meet the required standards of scholarship but also to ensure that your clinical, educational, and academic contributions are appropriately recognized.

Chapter 26
Obtaining Additional Degrees: When, Where, and How

Genevieve A. Fasano and Vivian J. Bea

Introduction

As surgeons, we are good at school. We need to be given how many years of schooling it takes to become a surgeon. Let's do the math. We start with four years of college to obtain an undergraduate degree, the prerequisite for medical school. Then, of course, there are four more years as a medical school student. At this point, even though we are technically doctors, wait, there is more to go—this time, in the form of residency. While residency can span anywhere from 2 to 7 years, for surgeons, it's usually on the upper limit of that range. Most of us pursue 5 or even 7 years of residency, depending on our chosen program. So why would any surgeon want to pursue even more years of schooling to obtain an additional degree?

The concept of dual-degree programs first became apparent when I realized I wanted to attend medical school. I realized that although I wanted to become a surgeon, there were additional opportunities for obtaining not just a medical degree, but also perhaps a Master of Public Health (MPH), Master of Business Administration (MBA)/Executive Masters of Business Administration (EMBA), Masters in Health Administration (MHA)/Executive in Health Administration (EMHA), or even a PhD.

But as surgeons, we are also excellent planners—we have to be, given the many balls we are often juggling. The importance of planning is paramount when you are considering pursuing an additional degree, since there are many opportunities during training to do so, including medical school. However, it does require additional

G. A. Fasano (✉)
Department of Surgery, Weill Cornell Medicine, New York, NY, USA
e-mail: vivianjbea@gmail.com

V. J. Bea (✉)
Section Chief of Breast Surgical Oncology, Department of Surgery, New York- Presbyterian Brooklyn Methodist Hospital, New York, NY, USA
e-mail: vjb9003@med.cornell.edu

K. Yoon-Flannery et al. (eds.), *Women in Surgery*,
https://doi.org/10.1007/978-3-032-10971-2_26

layers of planning the farther along we go. Take residency, for example. Most academic residency programs now have mandated or strongly suggested academic or research time. This includes 2 or 3 years in which your clinical duties are put aside so that you can focus on other aspects of career development. For most, this involves either clinical or basic science research. However, this also becomes an opportune time to obtain an additional degree (Figs. 26.1 and 26.2).

Let's say you've committed to 2 years of dedicated research, perhaps during residency. Many degree requirements heavily overlap with the work you may already be doing. You may consider a master's degree in epidemiology, health services, or outcomes research, or even an MPH. Now more than ever, there are many advanced degrees that complement surgical training (Table 26.1). For some, depending on the institution, many residents can also pursue these degrees within their institution's medical or graduate school. This can often lead to a seamless transition and the ability to collaborate with and be mentored by other faculty members within the institution that you would not interact with otherwise. In some cases, the institution may also offer discounted tuition rates or other means of sponsorship.

As an attending, taking on graduate school for an additional degree requires even more dedication and, as already noted, planning. Clinical responsibilities may need to be shifted, which requires buy-in from your institutional leadership. Additionally,

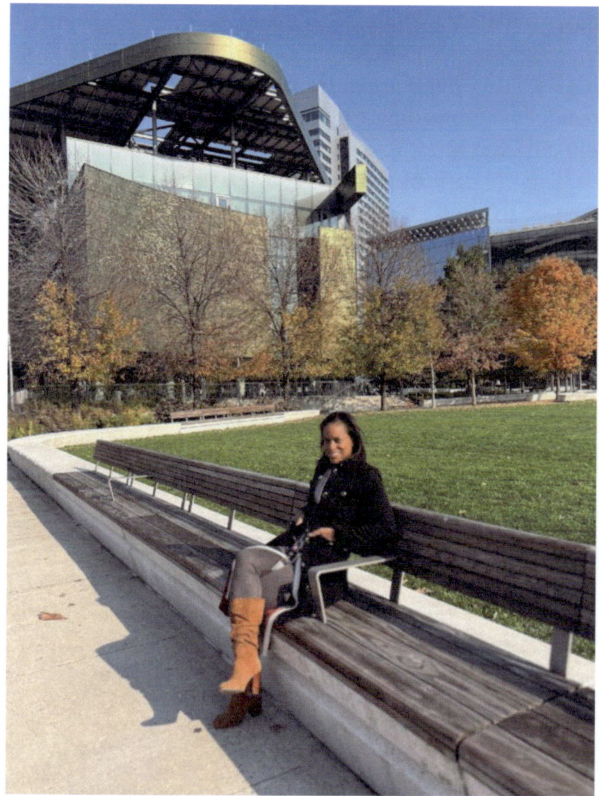

Fig. 26.1 Vivian Jolley Bea, MD Breast Surgical Oncologist at Cornell Tech attending Saturday EMBA/MS in healthcare classes at Cornell SC Johnson College of Business/Weill Cornell Medicine in New York

Fig. 26.2 Vivian J. Bea, MD pitching at Cornell University

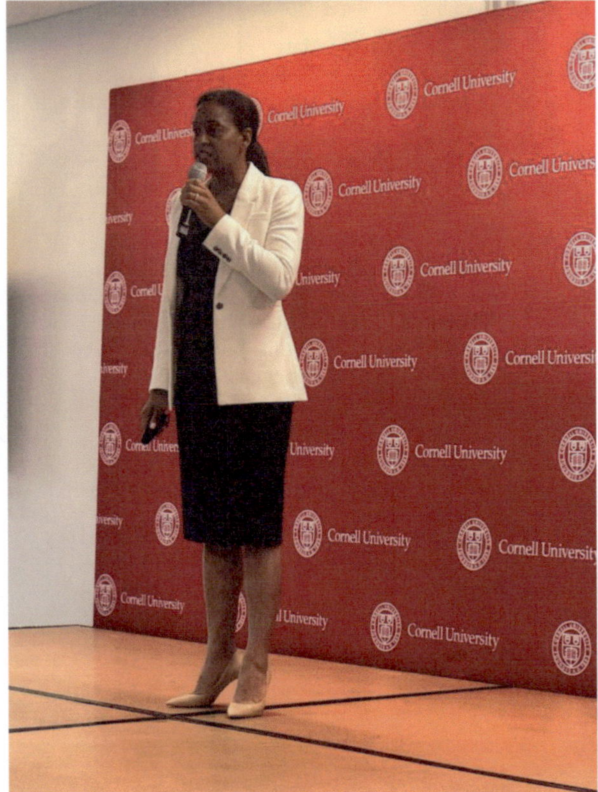

flexibility from the program that you are enrolled in is essential, as the time it takes to complete the degree may be longer than for other non-healthcare students, depending on your practice. It is also important to consider that at this point in our careers, many of us also have other responsibilities outside of the hospital, like a family and young children. Many programs account for these factors, such as an executive MBA and executive MHA, where coursework is done predominantly on nights and/or weekends.

As surgeons, we are lifelong learners, and for many, this is what drew us to this career in the first place. While there are various points in time to pursue additional degrees during training or during the early stages of a career, the benefits are wide-ranging. Networking with like-minded individuals both within and outside health-care often leads to multidisciplinary collaborations that may extend beyond the degree program. Obtaining an advanced degree can also empower you to take on new roles outside of classical clinical responsibilities, allowing for a more varied and fulfilling career. Offering new perspectives, programs can also provide the tools to shift a surgeon's career trajectory or take on new positions down the line (Fig. 26.3).

Table 26.1 Additional degrees for surgeons and expected length of training

Type of degree	Master's degree	Master of Business Administration (MBA/EMBA)	Master of Public Health (MPH)	Masters of Health Administration (MHA/EMHA)	Doctor of Philosophy (PhD)
Area of study	Clinical and Translational Investigation Clinical Epidemiology and Health Services Research Genetic Counseling Population Health Sciences Healthcare Leadership and Administration	Broad-based education in business management, strategic thinking, problem-solving, communication skills, and teamwork	Prepares students to work in public health by teaching epidemiology, environmental health, health policy, biostatistics, program planning, and best practices to address health issues	Prepares students to work in public health by teaching epidemiology, environmental health, health policy, biostatistics, program planning, and best practices to address health issues	Development of critical knowledge in a specific scientific area
Time to Complete[a]	1–2 years	1–2 years	1–2 years	1–2 years	3–5 years

[a]Note that the time to complete each degree is provided as an estimate, but may vary based on the individual and program

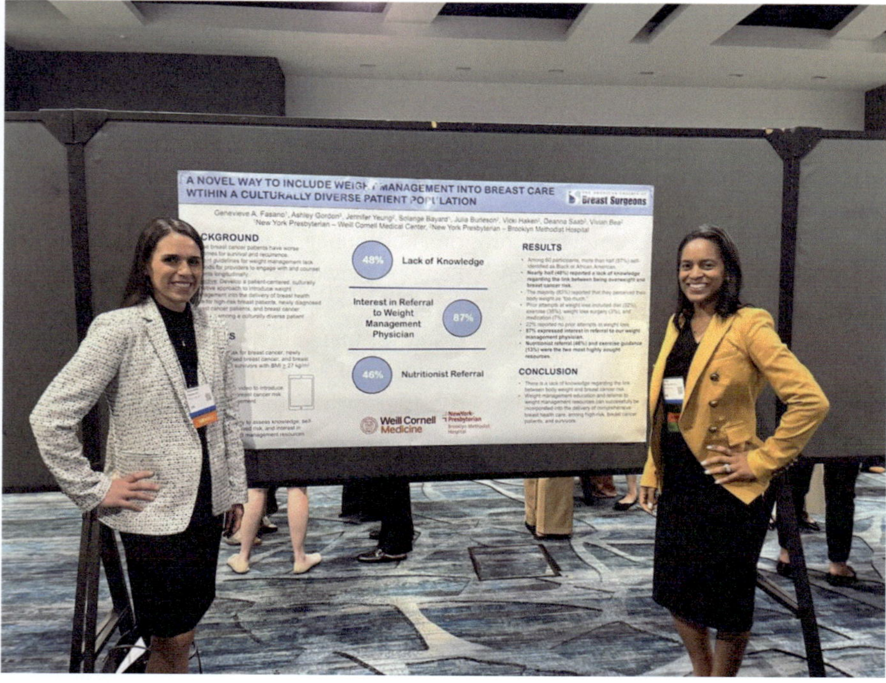

Fig. 26.3 Genevieve A. Fasano, MD and Vivian J. Bea, MD presenting research at the American Society of Breast Surgeons annual meeting

If you are contemplating obtaining an additional degree, here are some general recommendations:

1. Plan ahead

    (a) Utilize your excellent planning skills to determine early on what skillsets will be useful in your desired career, and what degree will provide the right training. For example, if clinical research will be a major component, consider a master's degree in clinical epidemiology, health services research, or clinical and translational investigation. If healthcare leadership is within your goals, consider an MBA/EMBA, MHA/EMBA, or a master's program with coursework that includes healthcare leadership, operations, management, and/or healthcare policy.

2. Find a mentor

    (a) Having a mentor to help navigate the process is vital. Talk to other surgeons who have advanced degrees to hear about their experience and how they made it work while balancing their clinical responsibilities. Learn from their experience.

3. Develop a financial strategy

    (a) As surgeons, we are all experienced in strategizing for the financial cost of higher education. Many surgical trainees and early to mid-career surgeons face large amounts of student debt; therefore, this step is essential. Determine early on how you will pay for the cost of the program. If pursuing a degree within your institution, inquire about discounted rates and options for tuition reimbursement or scholarships.

4. Be flexible

    (a) Recognize that your path toward whatever degree you pursue may not look like the other members of your cohort—and that is perfectly acceptable. Give yourself grace as you take on this additional role while continuing your responsibilities within your healthcare team and your patients.

Chapter 27
Promoting Gender Equity in Surgical Workplaces

Mckenzie Rowe and Paula Ferrada

Introduction

As a woman in surgery, I have witnessed both progress and persistent challenges in achieving gender equity. As of 2023-2024, women represent over half of medical students, nearly half (49%) of surgical residents, and approximately one quarter of active surgeons, with representation steadily increasing [2, 7]. Yet, when I walk into the operating room, I am often reminded that true gender equality has not been achieved.

The barriers women in surgery face are not always blatant but exist in the subtle, everyday interactions that shape our careers. For many of us, gender equity isn't about statistics— it's embedded in our daily interactions. *Are we given the same respect and opportunities as our male colleagues?* From the patient who assumes I am their nurse to the scheduling disparities that favor our male colleagues, these challenges accumulate, creating an environment where women must *constantly prove they belong*.

M. Rowe (✉)
Department of Surgery, Inova Fairfax Health, Falls Church, VA, USA
e-mail: Mckenzie.Rowe@inova.org

P. Ferrada
Department of Surgery Inova Fairfax Medical Campus, Falls Church, VA, USA

Medical Director Perioperative Services IFMC, Falls Church, VA, USA

Division and System Chief for Trauma and Acute Care Surgery Inova Healthcare System, Falls Church, VA, USA

University of Virginia School of Medicine, Charlottesville, VA, USA

ELAM class 2020, Falls Church, VA, USA
e-mail: Paula.Ferrada@inova.org

K. Yoon-Flannery et al. (eds.), *Women in Surgery*,
https://doi.org/10.1007/978-3-032-10971-2_27

Despite these obstacles, I have also witnessed the power of mentorship, sponsorship, and allyship in paving the way for meaningful change. I have seen institutions adapt policies to support pregnant surgeons, male colleagues advocate for fairer workplace structures, and national organizations push for systemic reforms. These efforts are making a difference, but there is still much work to be done.

For gender equity to become a reality in surgery, we must address the deeply ingrained biases and structural inequities that persist. This chapter explores the key areas where change is needed—mentorship and sponsorship, pregnancy and parental leave policies, implicit bias, operating room (OR) dynamics, acknowledgment of the confidence gap between men and women, and institutional reforms—offering solutions that can create a more inclusive and supportive surgical profession for all. Furthermore, it is critical to recognize that increasing gender equity in surgery is not just about fairness; research consistently shows that female surgeons have better patient outcomes, making gender equity a benefit to the entire field of surgery [10, 11].

Mentorship, Sponsorship, and Allyship

Mentorship has been a critical component of my success in surgery. As a student, I was told countless times—mostly by non-surgeons—that a surgical career would be incompatible with having a family. I was fortunate to have women surgeons at my institution who were open to meeting with me and served as examples of surgeons as mothers. They provided guidance, shared their experiences, and encouraged me to pursue my goals without compromise.

Beyond mentorship, *sponsorship* is equally important. A sponsor is someone who actively advocates for your career advancement by providing visibility and opportunities. It is key for us all to both find and be those mentors and sponsors for each other. It cannot be understated the importance of recommending other women for projects, committees, promotions, and speaking engagements. Even seemingly small actions, such as inviting a junior faculty member to a dinner with senior members, could be the stepping stone they need to grow or advance.

Allyship extends beyond mentorship and sponsorship. Men and other advocates in surgery play a vital role in promoting gender equity by actively recognizing and addressing disparities. Whether by advocating for equitable parental leave policies, ensuring women are included in leadership conversations, or calling out biases when they see them, allies play a crucial role in fostering change.

Pregnancy, Parental Leave, and Family Support

One of the most significant challenges for many women in surgery is *balancing professional and personal lives*, particularly parenting. We cannot ignore the clear societal pressure women experience to be the primary homemakers, caregivers, and the main node of emotional support within a home. The significant physical demands of pregnancy and breastfeeding add to an already burdensome workload for women at home and work, which takes a physical and emotional toll on women surgeons.

Women in surgery face a higher risk of pregnancy complications (discussed more in other chapters) due to long hours, high stress levels, physically demanding work, and delayed family planning [5]. At my institution, we implemented a *Pregnancy Curriculum* for residents, which includes structured accommodations such as scheduled breaks during long cases, excused prenatal visits, limiting radiation exposure, lactation facilities near the ORs, and flexible scheduling upon return [6]. These adjustments have significantly improved the experience for pregnant residents, demonstrating that institutional support can make a meaningful difference.

Historically, *parental leave* in surgery has carried a significant stigma, with many women feeling pressured to return to work quickly [4]. Though attitudes have improved, the tension between professional and personal responsibilities remains. Many women still experience guilt when prioritizing family over work—or vice versa—while societal and institutional biases often question their commitment [4, 8].

To create a truly equitable workplace, hospitals must provide comprehensive parental leave policies, allow pregnant surgeons in their third and fourth trimesters to modify their schedules, and offer affordable and flexible childcare options. Critically, *these benefits should extend to all parents*, regardless of gender, to help normalize caregiving responsibilities for everyone and reduce stigma for women.

Implicit Bias and Workplace Discrimination

Implicit bias and overt discrimination remain pervasive challenges for women surgeons. Society still associates men with being doctors and women with being nurses, leading to frequent misidentifications. I think we all have had countless experiences of being called a "nurse" despite introducing ourselves as someone's doctor. I've also been more likely to receive requests from patients for nonphysician tasks, such as fetching water, a boost in bed, or ordering a meal, compared to my male colleagues, reinforcing outdated stereotypes. While these are seemingly simple tasks, they add an extra burden that is far less expected from our male counterparts.

Bias extends beyond patient interactions to surgeons and other staff. Something that is not often said, but I think often felt, is that a lot of the bias and discrimination in the workplace actually comes from *other women*. Women surgeons more often receive both formal and informal complaints from female staff for being "aggressive" or "unprofessional" when displaying leadership traits that are accepted in men. Research shows that women surgeons are more likely to receive these complaints when responding in high-stakes situations where decisiveness is critical or performance-related issues in the OR [6]. This double standard forces many women to temper their assertiveness to avoid negative perceptions, contributing to stress and burnout.

Simple actions—such as consistently referring to female residents and attendings as "Dr." in front of patients and staff—reinforce respect and authority. Addressing incorrect assumptions and advocating for women in leadership roles further fosters a culture of equity and inclusion.

Gender Bias in the Operating Room

Gender disparities extend further into the OR, where scheduling practices often favor men surgeons. Studies have shown that, after controlling for specialty, men surgeons were significantly more likely to have overlapping cases, consecutive cases, shorter turnover times, and a greater number of cases per day [13]. In my experience, I have observed OR staff making greater efforts to accommodate male surgeons' preferences, while women who express frustration about delays are often labeled as "difficult." These time disparities could be a potential driver of inequities in professional outcomes, such as advancement or pay between surgeons by gender. Additionally, direct observation teamwork assessments reveal that women surgeons receive less frequent updates from OR staff, which could impact their ability to manage cases effectively [3]. These interprofessional conflicts can impact women emotionally, professionally, and cause delays in patient care.

These inequities highlight the need for institutional recognition of gender biases in OR culture, logistics, and scheduling. Standardized scheduling policies and regular bias training for OR staff could help mitigate these disparities. Organizations such as the Association of Women Surgeons (AWS) have proposed strategies, including committing to a culture shift, introducing bias literacy, encouraging sponsorship, and promoting deliberative decision-making in hiring and promotions [1].

Adapting Teaching Styles for Gender Differences

Surgical education must evolve to recognize and address differences in how men and women approach learning and self-assessment. Research consistently shows that, despite performing equally on objective measures, women medical students and surgical residents report lower confidence than their male counterparts [9]. In the field of surgery, where confidence is often equated with competence, this disparity can have real consequences—limiting autonomy, slowing advancement, and shaping how educators perceive female trainees.

I have experienced both ends of the spectrum in responses from attendings when I ask questions—those who recognize this as a reflection of thoroughness and push me to trust what I already know, and others who interpret my questions as a lack of ability. The latter approach can be damaging, reinforcing doubts on both sides rather than building confidence.

As educators and leaders, we need to recognize that confidence and competence are not the same. Women may ask more clarifying questions—not because they lack knowledge, but because they want certainty before acting. Instead of interpreting this as hesitation or weakness, educators should use it as an opportunity to foster growth for both trainees and faculty. Encouraging calculated risk-taking, reinforcing what learners already know, and ensuring women receive the same level of autonomy as their male colleagues are key steps in closing this gap. Faculty development should address these differences explicitly, ensuring that teaching methods empower, rather than sideline, female trainees and faculty.

Institutional- and National-Level Change

While individual efforts are critical, lasting change requires institutional- and national-level interventions. Hospitals must adopt unbiased hiring practices, promote pay transparency, implement strong parental leave policies, and address implicit bias. National organizations like AWS, the American College of Surgeons (ACS), and Gender Equity Initiative in Global Surgery (GEIGS) play a crucial role in providing resources to both individuals and institutions on how to make these changes. These groups provide mentorship programs, develop bias training, advocate for policy reform, raise awareness, and support research to advance industry standards. Recent progress can be seen last year with statements by the ACS and ABS, such as their recommendation for a minimum of 6 weeks of postpartum leave, no make-up call from leave, and RVU adjustments. These represent a positive step, but further improvements are needed to ensure true equity [12].

Conclusion: Moving Forward

The path to gender equity in surgery is ongoing, but meaningful change is within reach. By fostering mentorship and sponsorship, advocating for family-friendly policies, addressing implicit bias, and pushing for institutional reforms, we can create a more inclusive and supportive surgical profession.

Gender equity is not just about fairness—it strengthens the field as a whole. When all surgeons, regardless of gender, are valued and supported, patient outcomes improve, workplace cultures thrive, and the profession becomes more sustainable. It is the responsibility of individuals, institutions, and national organizations to ensure that the next generation of surgeons enters a profession that truly upholds equity, respect, and opportunity for all.

References

1. DiBrito, S. R., Lopez, C. M., Jones, C., & Mathur, A. (2019). Reducing Implicit Bias: Association of Women Surgeons #HeForShe Taskforce Best Practices Recommendations. *Journal of the American College of Surgeons*, *228*(3), 303–309. https://doi.org/10.1016/j.jamcollsurg.2018.12.011

2. Haskins, J. (2019, July 15). Where are all the women in surgery? *AAMC*. https://www.aamc.org/news/where-are-all-women-surgery

3. Jonas, N., Bourgeois, D., Zahira, T. et al. (2022). *Unexpected findings of gender bias after a correlation of operating room teamwork assessment tools.* https://doi.org/10.1007/s44186-022-00086-1

4. *Parental Leave.* (2022, January 3). [Broadcast]. https://open.spotify.com/show/0tSNVnjep1pA1qMGLEoEsa

5. Rangel, E. L., Castillo-Angeles, M., Easter, S. R., Atkinson, R. B., Gosain, A., Hu, Y.-Y., Cooper, Z., Dey, T., & Kim, E. (2021). Incidence of Infertility and Pregnancy Complications in US Female Surgeons. *JAMA Surgery*, *156*(10), 905–915. https://doi.org/10.1001/jamasurg.2021.3301

6. Sterbling, H. M., Kelly, C. H., Stafford, A., Willey, S., & Dort, J. (2023). Pregnancy Curriculum: Advocating for a Healthier Pregnancy in General Surgery Residency. *Journal of Surgical Education*, *80*(12), 1799–1805. https://doi.org/10.1016/j.jsurg.2023.08.004

7. *Table B3. Number of Active Residents, by Type of Medical School, GME Specialty, and Gender.* (2024, October 14). AAMC. https://www.aamc.org/data-reports/students-residents/data/report-residents/2024/table-b3-number-active-residents-type-medical-school-gme-specialty-and-gender

8. Torres, A. J. C., Barbosa-Silva, L., Oliveira-Silva, L. C., Miziara, O. P. P., Guahy, U. C. R., Fisher, A. N., & Ryan, M. K. (2024). The Impact of Motherhood on Women's Career Progression: A Scoping Review of Evidence-Based Interventions. *Behavioral Sciences*, *14*(4), Article 4. https://doi.org/10.3390/bs14040275

9. Van Boerum, M. S., Jarman, A. F., Veith, J., McCarty Allen, C., Holoyda, K. A., Agarwal, C., Crombie, C., & Cochran, A. (2020). The confidence gap: Findings for women in plastic surgery. *The American Journal of Surgery*, *220*(5), 1351–1357. https://doi.org/10.1016/j.amjsurg.2020.06.037

10. Wallis, C. J. D., Jerath, A., Aminoltejari, K., Kaneshwaran, K., Salles, A., Coburn, N., Wright, F. C., Gotlib Conn, L., Klaassen, Z., Luckenbaugh, A. N., Ranganathan, S., Riveros, C., McCartney, C., Armstrong, K., Bass, B., Detsky, A. S., & Satkunasivam, R. (2023). Surgeon Sex and Long-Term Postoperative Outcomes Among Patients Undergoing Common Surgeries. *JAMA Surgery*, *158*(11), 1185–1194. https://doi.org/10.1001/jamasurg.2023.3744

11. Wallis, C. J., Ravi, B., Coburn, N., Nam, R. K., Detsky, A. S., & Satkunasivam, R. (2017). Comparison of postoperative outcomes among patients treated by male and female surgeons: A population based matched cohort study. *The BMJ*, *359*, j4366. https://doi.org/10.1136/bmj.j4366

12. *Workplace Support for Practicing Surgeons | ABS.* (2024). American Board of Surgery. https://www.absurgery.org/resources/news/workplace-support-practicing-surgeons/

13. Wright, K., Hamilton, K., & Friedman, J. (2024). Novel metrics to measure gender bias in operating room scheduling priority. *American Journal of Obstetrics & Gynecology*, *230*(6), e117–e120. https://doi.org/10.1016/j.ajog.2024.01.025

Chapter 28
Advocacy Efforts for Women in Training and Practice

Stephanie Bonne

Advocacy can come in many forms, and surgeons are well poised to be excellent advocates. Many women have been advocates their entire lives, even if we don't realize it. Women often advocated for themselves as girls, to be included, or have their voice heard in science and math classes where implicit, or at times, explicit bias put them at a disadvantage compared to their male peers. Many of us volunteered or participated in social causes or movements in young adulthood, advocating for people without a voice or who had less agency in society than ourselves. And as physicians, we advocate for ourselves and our patients every day.

As daily advocates for ourselves and our patients, it's a natural extension to advance into more structured advocacy work. Advocacy work can be institutional, such as advocating for resources, programs, or support for a project or program we are passionate about. It may be advocating institutionally for resources for another person or a group of individuals, such as advocating for students who want to form a new student organization.

Advocacy may also be political or public advocacy. This comes in the form of advocating for groups of people who need money, policy change, or attention and resources in order to accomplish a particular goal. Surgical organizations may participate in structured political advocacy efforts to advance the goals of their members or advance the agenda of the organization. Coalitions may advocate for a policy change that will allow easier access to resources for the people they serve [1, 2].

If you find a cause or issue that you want to advocate for, there are some considerations to guide your efforts, and some questions you should ask yourself as you prepare your advocacy efforts.

S. Bonne (✉)
Professor of Surgery, Wake Forest University School of Medicine, Winston-Salem, NC, USA

Department of Surgery, Advocate Christ Medical Center, Oak Lawn, IL, USA
e-mail: Stephanie.bonne@aah.org

K. Yoon-Flannery et al. (eds.), *Women in Surgery*,
https://doi.org/10.1007/978-3-032-10971-2_28

1. Is this effort relevant to my work as a surgeon, or is this an individual issue? For example, advocating for funding for your local library is probably best approached as an individual effort, whereas advocating for funding for a surgical simulator for your residents would clearly benefit from your voice as a surgeon. Advocating for scholarships for women in STEM careers could be both personal and professional.

2. Understand how using your voice in your professional capacity could affect your employment, and have discussions about the appropriateness of your involvement in your advocacy effort with your employer. You should do this even in innocuous conditions. For example, perhaps you want to advocate for a community garden in a vacant parcel of land near your hospital. Sounds simple enough, right? But maybe, unknown to you, your hospital is looking to purchase that property to build a clinic space, and this is controversial among the community members. You have just put yourself in the middle of a hot-button issue between the community and the hospital, and could potentially be dragged into some contentious social media.

3. Find other stakeholders and partners in your effort. This could take a long time and a lot of effort, depending on what you are trying to advocate for. Perhaps you want to advocate for increased funding for your state's trauma system. Your single voice in your statehouse may hold some weight, but not nearly as much weight as a group of community coalitions, the hospital association, and other major medical groups going as a single voice. Developing these coalitions and organizing together may be more helpful. Additionally, other coalition members may help you identify pitfalls or help you understand nuances related to your issue.

4. If your issue involves you interacting with either media or politicians, seek out help from your institution's media and government relations offices. All major medical centers and universities have offices that support the priorities of their institutions in government and respond to the media. These individuals can help make sure you are representing your institution in a way that is consistent with their messaging and help you avoid any pitfalls or missteps in your advocacy effort. They can also help coach you for social media, help you write op-eds, or help you prepare for radio or television interviews.

5. Finally, seek out your societies and explain your priorities to them. Surgical societies are sometimes held up by 501c3 status that prohibits lobbying. However, the prohibition on lobbying does not prohibit advocacy or speaking out on particular issues. Many societies will have an associated PAC that is a separate entity for lobbying and funding political campaigns. Societies should listen to their members about what issues should be addressed by their advocacy committees, and may listen if you bring an issue forward that you are passionate about. You may find other like-minded individuals in your society who are eager to advocate for the same issue.

If you want to learn more about political advocacy and don't know where to get started, there are a plethora of resources available from surgical societies [1–3].

Being involved in state and local chapters of your society allows you to influence decisions that are being made at the state and local levels. Many organizations hold "hill days" in which you attend some preparation time and then go to Capitol Hill in Washington, DC, to meet with senators and representatives. These can be incredible learning experiences to shape your understanding of the legislative process, the accessibility of your representatives, and how to interact with their health policy staff and advisors. You can also set up meetings in your district with your representatives [4].

There are tips about meeting with representatives, whether they are political or an institutional leader, when advocating for a cause you care about. It is absolutely imperative to make sure you have a specific ask. Rather than asking someone to "support women in surgery," you might ask for a study on gender equity to be conducted by your organization. Perhaps you care about a legislative advocacy issue. You can look up pending legislation on the issue and ask your representative to cosponsor a forthcoming bill, or volunteer to write new legislation on the issue. You can ask them to vote in a specific way on a bill [5, 6].

It is also important that you understand and frame your ask in terms of the cost and benefit of the ask. If you are asking for a new program in your university, you should come armed with a budget and explain the advantages, where the money will come from, and how it will contribute either to future finances or to the mission of the institution. You may have data that supports the implementation of a program that was successful in another state, which you can take to your state legislators. Or you may be able to demonstrate that a vote on a certain bill will be very popular in a representative's district. Explaining why this is important to you, including your personal stories, but also painting the picture and showing that you understand the pitfalls and how to avoid them, can help your cause.

In short, women are incredible advocates for ourselves, for our profession, and for the causes that move us. Polishing our advocacy skills and building coalitions serves to strengthen our voices and makes us unstoppable forces for good in our profession and in the world around us.

References

1. American College of Surgeons State Advocacy Toolkit. Available at: http://acs-state-advocacy-toolkit.pdf
2. American College of Surgeons. How to Be a Surgeon Advocate. Available at: http://acs-state-advocacy-toolkit.pdf
3. The American Medical Association. Healthcare Advocacy. Available at: Health Care Advocacy | Physician Advocacy in Medicine | AMA
4. Liebe HL, Buonpane C, Lewis S, Golubkova A, Leiva T, Phillips R, Stewart K, Reinschmidt KM, Garwe T, Sarwar Z, Hunter CJ. This is Our Lane: A Pilot Study Examining the Surgeon's Role in Social Justice Advocacy. Am J Surg. 2022 Jan;223(1):194–200. doi: https://doi.org/10.1016/j.amjsurg.2021.08.041. Epub 2021 Sep 23. PMID: 34588129; PMCID: PMC9526451.

5. Lefever D, Kelly PD, Zuckerman SL, Agarwal N, Guthikonda B, Kimmell KT, Schirmer C, Rosenow JM, Cozzens J, Orrico KO, Menger R. Advocacy to Government and Stakeholders. World Neurosurg. 2021 Jul;151:380–385. doi: https://doi.org/10.1016/j.wneu.2021.01.129. Epub 2021 Feb 3. PMID: 33548536.
6. Fernandez Lynch H, Bateman-House A, Rivera SM. Academic Advocacy: Opportunities to Influence Health and Science Policy Under U.S. Lobbying Law. Acad Med. 2020 Jan;95(1):44–51. doi: https://doi.org/10.1097/ACM.0000000000003037. PMID: 31599758.

Chapter 29
Surgeons as Health System Leaders

Nicole Fox

Introduction

Historically, the pathway to success in academic surgery was narrowly defined. Surgeons were expected to excel clinically, be outstanding educators, and conduct high-quality research. Achievement in these areas produced what is referred to as the "triple threat." It was the formula resulting in academic promotion and ascension into leadership positions typically offered to surgeons, such as division head, department chair, or dean of a medical school. The number of papers published, grants received, or leadership positions held were markers of success as an academic surgeon. This narrow definition had the potential to limit opportunities for individuals who possessed interest and/or skills in other areas, such as finance, administration, quality, or patient safety, to name a few.

Fortunately, the climate, culture, and definition of "success" in academic surgery are changing. This is the result of a number of factors related to the rapidly evolving landscape of health care delivery. Dimick and colleagues articulated this well in an ASA Presidential session entitled "Navigating the Collision of Corporate Medicine and Changing Workforce Expectations." Session participants eloquently described the difficult reality of trying to preserve excellence in academic surgery in the face of increasing productivity demands and the need to tightly control labor expenses [1]. This is coupled with a changing workforce in which the next generation of surgeons is drawing strict boundaries and challenging the status quo. Although this may seem overwhelming, it presents the opportunity to redefine "leadership" and

N. Fox (✉)
Professor of Surgery, Associate Chief Medical Officer, Cooper Medical School of Rowan University, Camden, NJ, USA

Cooper University Health Care, Camden, NJ, USA
e-mail: fox-nicole@cooperhealth.edu

K. Yoon-Flannery et al. (eds.), *Women in Surgery*,
https://doi.org/10.1007/978-3-032-10971-2_29

"success" in academic surgery and highlight the different paths that surgeons can take to lead, effect change, and influence the shape of healthcare.

Defining Leadership

In his *TEDx Talk "How great leaders inspire action,"* Simon Sinek states that "leadership is a choice, not a rank. Anyone in an organization can be a leader. It's choosing to look out for the person on your left and to look out for the person on your right" [2]. At the most basic level, leadership requires an individual to look after others and commit time and effort to helping them succeed. Considering this definition, surgeons are well prepared to assume leadership roles. By virtue of their training, they understand how to lead a team in the operating room or at the bedside with the primary goal of alleviating suffering and disease. They advocate for patients and members of the clinical team on a daily basis. Surgeons interact with other specialists in delivering care and navigate complex challenges in nonclinical areas such as scheduling, supply-chain management, and quality control. They are viewed institutionally as leaders by clinical and nonclinical team members and are a valued member of the healthcare ecosystem.

Surgeons have a strong clinical foundation and perspective that traditional administrative leaders in healthcare do not. In their daily work, they perform a number of functions that are essential to effective leadership at the system level. Surgeons are in charge of diverse teams in the operating room, managing a variety of personalities and needs to achieve a common goal. They are keenly aware of the importance of maintaining high-quality and safety standards and strategies for doing so. They are accustomed to navigating complex systems and making rapid decisions under intense pressure. These unique strengths can be leveraged and maximized in nonsurgical leadership roles.

Challenges and Opportunities

Along with an appreciation of the fundamental strengths that surgeons possess, an honest appraisal of opportunities for surgeon leaders is critical. Specific challenges exist as surgeons move into leadership positions outside of their clinical roles. Intensity, perfectionism, and the ability to make rapid decisions with little information are required to succeed in the operating room. It becomes ingrained during surgical training and may result in a difficult transition outside of the OR. In addition, surgeons are perceived as intimidating, which can unknowingly impact interactions with non-surgeons. This does not mean to imply that surgeons cannot be successful in leadership roles outside of their clinical domain. Transitioning to a health system leadership role requires recognition of these challenges along with skill development in areas such as conflict management, communication, and negotiation. As Peters et al. eloquently pointed out, "the ability to converse fluently in both clinical and administrative worlds is critical to success. Surgical leaders are required to be exemplary in terms of clinical competencies, to demonstrate their knowledge of the world of surgery and validate their opinions. Leadership positions (outside of surgery) will then be seen as an *extra level of accomplishment, rather than a substitute for lack of clinical skills*. When co-workers see that a surgeon is able to successfully navigate multiple arenas, they are more likely to trust in a surgeon's ability to lead" [3].

A perceived challenge for surgeons is the fact that pursuing a broader leadership role in healthcare will result in less time spent in the operating room. One concern is that less time operating will result in "skill erosion." Whether or not this is perception or reality is multi-factorial and depends in part on the individual skill of the surgeon, the number of years in practice, and the willingness to be realistic about what they are able to contribute clinically. Balancing clinical responsibilities along with a system leadership role will require careful consideration and discussion with colleagues and department/division leadership. It will also require honest self-evaluation and solicitation of feedback on an ongoing basis. This is an area in which surgeons must be particularly vigilant.

Acquiring Additional Skills

There is no "set" curriculum for acquiring needed skills, and surgeons committed to leadership development must determine the method that works best for them. A number of options exist. For example, some choose to pursue an advanced degree such as a master's in business administration (MBA), master's in public health (MPH), or a master's in medical management (MMM). Professional organizations can provide an avenue for leadership development. The American College of Surgeons (ACS) offers a number of resources, including an annual leadership and advocacy summit, as well as scholarships, awards, and fellowship opportunities [4]. Subspecialty societies may offer leadership workshops or certificate programs. The American Association for Physician Leadership (AAPL) is well-established and has programs that are designed for physician leaders. Some hospitals have partnered with organizations like AAPL to run institution-specific leadership development programs for their faculty. An alternative to obtaining an advanced degree (which can be costly and time-intensive) is a certificate program, such as the certified physician executive (CPE) and/or executive leadership programs for physicians, offered through a number of universities [5, 6].

Training for surgeon leaders is not one-size-fits-all. The decision of what advanced training to pursue (if any) is highly individualized and should be carefully considered based on factors including overall goals, clinical workload, and financial feasibility. It is critical to research the numerous options available and identify (through self-evaluation) the specific skills one needs to develop as a leader.

Specific Roles to Consider

Healthcare organizations vary in the types of leadership opportunities that are available to physicians. In this section, the scope of some common roles is defined. This list is not all-encompassing and only intended to provide examples of system-level roles that may be of interest to surgeons. The existence of these roles may vary depending on the administrative structure of the organization and the type of health system (academic, community, etc.). There will not be a dedicated discussion of the Chief Executive Officer (CEO) role here. It is interesting to note that in a 2019 review of the topic of physician CEOs, Gupta reported that "since 1935, the number of hospitals managed by chief executive officers (CEOs) who are also physicians has decreased by 90%. Today, only 5% of hospitals in the United States are run by CEOs with a medical degree" [7]. Despite the uncommon occurrence of physician CEOs, those who inhabit this role run some of the best-performing hospitals in the United States [8]. A growing body of literature suggests that hospitals with physician executives outperform those without, and the unique perspective that physicians have from their clinical work is the key to that success.

A *chief physician executive (CPE)* is defined as "a senior-level healthcare leader who is a licensed physician, responsible for overseeing the medical operations of a healthcare organization while also managing the business aspects, essentially acting as a bridge between clinical practice and administrative leadership within the organization." Not every hospital has a CPE; however, the role has become more visible over the last 5–10 years. The CPE participates in strategic planning, budgeting, and management of the physician practice. They generally serve as the primary liaison between the medical staff and hospital administration to ensure that clinical operations align with organizational goals.

A *chief medical officer (CMO)* commonly serves as the highest-ranking physician executive in a hospital (particularly those hospitals that do not have a CPE role). The CMO position is a "dual role," meaning that these are established physician leaders who work clinically and are also members of the executive leadership team. Some typical responsibilities of a CMO include, but are not limited to, performing needs assessments for the organization, ensuring compliance with federal/state laws and safety regulations, working with department chairs to set budgets and determine equipment needs, and managing the physician practice, including professionalism issues that require disciplinary action. The CMO role may be more palatable for surgeons because it allows them to maintain a clinical practice (limited) and lead within the health system.

A *vice-president of medical affairs (VPMA)* is a senior executive who typically reports to the CMO of the hospital. Although the responsibilities of this role may vary by organization and overlap with the duties of the CMO, this individual will drive quality improvement initiatives, manage physician relations, ensure compliance with healthcare regulations, and work closely with the executive team to achieve strategic goals for the hospital while ensuring high-quality care and maintaining physician engagement. It is not clear how many hospitals have CMO and/or

VPMA roles or both. A survey conducted in 2009 indicated "when asked if the role of CMO or VPMA exists in their organizations, 66% of respondents cite having a CMO, 43% cite having a VPMA, and 26% confirm that both roles are present in their organization" [9].

CEO, CPE, CMO, and VPMA positions are well-established roles in the health system that can (or must) be occupied by physicians. It is important to keep in mind that there are a host of leadership roles outside of the C-suite that are appropriate for surgeons and would enable them to make a difference in health care beyond their clinical role. Departments such as quality and safety, medical informatics, infection prevention, clinical documentation, and others have recognized the strength of having a physician (particularly a surgeon) leader in their department. This has resulted in the creation of roles at many hospitals, such as Medical Director of Quality, Patient Safety Officer, Chief Medical Informatics Officer, and Medical Director of Clinical Documentation Integrity, just to name a few. These are opportunities for surgeons to get involved and receive on-the-job training in management, finance, and hospital operations. Early, smaller leadership roles may ultimately set physicians on the path to higher-level system leadership and should be seriously considered and evaluated when offered.

Conclusion

For most surgeons, career success will continue to be defined by achievements in their chosen specialty and movement into traditional surgical leadership positions such as division head, department chair, or chief of staff. Yet, it is clear that the skill set surgeons possess and the wealth of clinical experience they offer is unique and lends itself well to broader leadership roles. The purpose of this chapter was to acknowledge that surgeons are valuable leaders at the system level. The information is intended for surgeons who "think they have an interest in health care beyond practicing surgery and taking care of patients clinically every day. Individuals who would like to make a big impact on how system-wide health care is delivered" [10]. In 2019, Dr. Barbara Bass reflected on surgical leadership in changing times. She stated that "the modern form of surgeon leadership empowerment is a responsibility to serve as a collaborative leader of high-performance teams" [11]. Ideally, increasing numbers of surgeons will explore unconventional leadership paths in medicine and work to drive system-level change.

References

1. Dimick J., Harris C., Barrett M., Kent K., Sosa JA. and Farmer D. (2023). Navigating the collision of corporate medicine and changing workforce expectations. *Annals of Surgery*, 278 (4), 471–78.

2. TED (2010, May 4). *How great leaders inspire action* (Video). YouTube. https://www.youtube.com/watch?v=qp0HIF3SfI4
3. Peters W., Picchioni A., Fleshman J. (2020). Surgical leadership. *Cln Colon Rectal Surg*, 33, 233–37.
4. https://www.facs.org/for-medical-professionals/conferences-and-meetings/leadership-and-advocacy-summit/Aapl.org
5. https://www.physicianleaders.org/
6. https://professional.dce.harvard.edu/find-a-program/
7. Gupta A. (2019). Physician versus non-physician CEOs: the effect of a leader's background on the quality of hospital management and healthcare. *Journal of Hospital Administration*, 8(5), 47–51.
8. Goodall AH (2011). Physician leaders and hospital performance: is there an association? *Soc Sci Med*, 73(4), 535–539.
9. Dister L. (2009). CMO or VPMA-is there a difference? *Physician Executive*, 35(3), 12.
10. Shoup M. (2019). Central surgical association presidential address: top ten reasons surgeons make great health care leaders. *Surgery*, 166, 431–34.
11. Bass BL. (2019). Surgical leadership in changing times: the American College of Surgeons perspective. *Innov Surg Sci*, 4(2), 75–83.

Chapter 30
Directing a Fellowship

Betty Fan and Carla Suzanne Fisher

Introduction

Directing a surgical fellowship program can be a fulfilling and influential position. A fellowship program acts not only as a training environment for upcoming leaders in the field but also allows the program to shape the future in their specialty. A well-run fellowship program will boost an institution's reputation and exposure. Serving in a program director role directly allows for the opportunity to become a lifelong mentor and role model for many physicians in their training program. Furthermore, the position of a fellowship director can provide increased exposure to prominent and senior members in your field as well as meaningful engagement in specialty societies.

Running a successful fellowship program has its own set of challenges. Ultimately, it requires a delicate balance focused on prioritizing the integrity of the fellowship training program as well as the needs of each individual fellow who chooses to train at your program. Like any endeavor of this magnitude, it requires time and effort that can be difficult to work within a busy surgeon's schedule.

The establishment of a successful fellowship training program and maintaining its standing falls largely on the efforts of the program director. With a brand new or early program, garnering leadership support at your institution to commit to the requirements and resources needed to run a fellowship program is often the first step. This will often require showing the merits of having a fellowship at the

B. Fan (✉)
Breast Surgery, Department of General Surgery, University of Chicago, Chicago, IL, USA
e-mail: fanb@uchicagomedicine.org

C. S. Fisher
Professor of Surgery, Chief, Division of Breast Surgery, Indiana University School of Medicine, Indianapolis, IN, USA
e-mail: fishercs@iu.edu

K. Yoon-Flannery et al. (eds.), *Women in Surgery*,
https://doi.org/10.1007/978-3-032-10971-2_30

institution as well as the financial sustainability of the program. Some fellowships will allow fellows to bill independently, and this is an important point to clarify for your program. When allowed and appropriate, this helps to offset the costs of maintaining the program. Funding of the fellowship can come from multiple sources, including your department, division, cancer center, philanthropic, or even industry support. The source will certainly be affected by institutional guidelines, and it's important to understand how the funding works, as it can change and potentially compromise your ability to offer training positions.

Like any training program, there are requirements for the fellows, but also for the program and the program director. For instance, some of the governing bodies require that the director be in clinical practice, following a fellowship, for a certain period of time prior to serving in this role. The exact requirements of each fellowship program differ and are beyond the scope of this chapter. However, similar principles apply broadly for all directors, including recruitment and engagement of dedicated teaching faculty and coordination amongst other departments required for the fellowship curriculum. The importance of a team of physician staff committed to fellow learning cannot be overemphasized, as they can help share in the demands of the teaching curriculum and reflect positively on the fellowship's reputation. This often provides an opportunity for the fellowship director to interact and engage with other faculty members.

An often overlooked but critical team member for a fellowship is the fellowship coordinator. Depending on the institution and size of the program, sometimes this is covered by an administrative assistant, but often this individual is housed within a dedicated education group. A fellowship coordinator is essential and will offload significant tasks, including scheduling burdens, documentation requirements, and program organization, from the program director, allowing them to focus on bigger picture items.

The program director has a significant role in the reputation and culture of the fellowship. This depends heavily on the environment and examples they choose to cultivate. Graduates serve as spokespeople of the fellowship and evidence of a strong training program. While keeping in mind the requirements set forth by the governing bodies for fellowships, equally important is identifying and adapting to the learning styles of each fellow recruited yearly. As the program director, adjusting to the personalities as well as strengths and weaknesses of each fellow they train contributes heavily to the success of the program. Common challenges program directors encounter include motivating individuals who may be suffering from burnout from being in training for years already, as well as those who may have other stressors on their minds, such as board exams and job searching. Finding each individual fellow's interest and passion may be one method of encouraging an engaged learner while also meeting the requirements of the fellowship. Building trust and rapport as a mentor early on can also serve to create a fulfilling fellowship relationship. Identifying future job goals is important to do with your fellow early on in the fellowship.

Mixed challenges exist for program directors depending on their own standing in their career timeline. It's important to note that there is no "perfect time" to take on the role of fellowship director. As noted earlier, this may depend on requirements by the governing body, but there are many other factors that affect when you might take on this role. For more early-career program directors, finding a balance of growing your own clinical and/or academic career and this role can be difficult. In contrast, your closeness to the trainee's side of training can be a positive. It can make it easier to see issues from the learner's perspective and promote a trainee-focused learning environment. One example may be as it relates to job-searching. Having likely been searching for a job not that long ago compared to your current fellow, an early-career program director may provide important insight into the current hiring environment, as well as provide up-to-date networking connections that can be valuable for your fellow. Conversely, program directors further along in their careers can benefit from the knowledge of experience as well as their own lessons from trial and errors in the past. Importantly, this role must be able to fit into your current responsibilities. Your own mentors or previous program directors should be able to provide some guidance on the time required and the best ways to integrate into your schedule. Some programs have Associate Program Director roles that provide a good transition into this role. Along these lines, will you be compensated in any way for this role? Like many academic roles, this is not always an area where you will see direct financial reward, but there are other ways your time can be compensated, and this should be investigated. Again, this also depends on the size of your program and overall fellowship requirements.

Successful recruitment and graduation of fellows can often be a large stressor for program directors. Newer fellowship programs may need to be flexible and more strategic in their interviewing and match process to increase their chances of a successful match. Ensuring fellows graduate consistently and obtain sought-after jobs can also further promote the desirability of the program. As fellowship programs evolve, the selection process for the fellowship director may shift towards recruiting fellows who more closely align with the vision of the program. When a fellowship program becomes more successful and therefore more competitive, the selectivity during the recruiting process may change as more applicants compete for the same position. Fellowship directors then must determine the direction they want to see their program shape into as their applicant pool increases (Fig. 30.1).

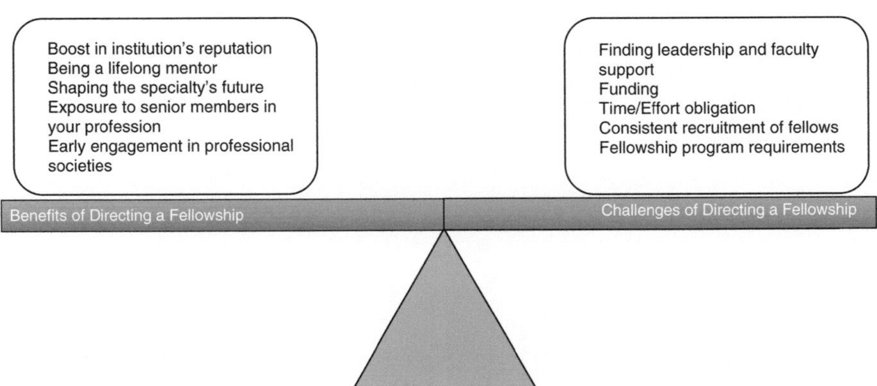

Fig. 30.1 Balancing a successful fellowship program

Conclusion

Ultimately, directing a fellowship program can be as rewarding as it is demanding. Attention to evolving teaching requirements of the fellowship program as well as the individualized needs of the fellows a program director mentors in their career remains the cornerstone of a successful program. Like many academic and leadership endeavors, developing a robust and supportive team can make the responsibilities of directing a fellowship easier and ensures a successful and lasting fellowship program.

Chapter 31
Being the President of a Society

Julie A. Margenthaler

Serving as the President of the American Society of Breast Surgeons was truly one of the most rewarding experiences I have had in my professional career. It represented the culmination of years of service in the society in a variety of roles that provided me with a great deal of insight regarding the importance of national societies and the mission they fulfill. As I reflect on that time, I have a better appreciation of the challenges and triumphs of that year and the impact that it had on my leadership style. I also recognize that it is a role that has not always been equitably filled by women surgeons.

Being a woman surgeon comes with numerous challenges, both professional and personal [1–3]. For many years, surgery has been a male-dominated field, which can manifest in unequal opportunities for advancement, disparities in salary, and a lack of mentorship from senior colleagues. Historically, this has extended to the national surgical societies as well. Only 21% of general surgeons are women, and certain subspecialties, such as orthopedics, remain predominantly male [4]. I am perhaps a more fortunate woman surgeon in the sense that I practice in a very woman-friendly surgical specialty. In the 27-year history of the American Society of Breast Surgeons, there have been 11 female presidents of the society [5]. In contrast, it was not until 2022 that Dr. Yolonda Colson became the first female President of the American Association for Thoracic Surgery [6] and Dr. Suzanne Klimberg became the first female President of the Southern Surgical Association [7], societies with 103 and 134 years of history, respectively. The American Academy of Orthopaedic Surgeons was founded in 1933; Dr. Kristy Weber was the first, and only, female president in 2019 [8]. Despite increased awareness of these challenges, systemic barriers and cultural attitudes persist, making it essential for women surgeons who have attained

J. A. Margenthaler (✉)
Professor of Surgery, Division of General Surgery, Section of Surgical Oncology,
Washington University in St. Louis, St. Louis, MO, USA
e-mail: jmargenthaler@wustl.edu

K. Yoon-Flannery et al. (eds.), *Women in Surgery*,
https://doi.org/10.1007/978-3-032-10971-2_31

leadership roles in national societies to continue to advocate for one another and support policies that enhance the representation and success of our female colleagues.

Becoming the president of a surgical society requires a combination of professional experience, leadership skills, and a demonstrated commitment to the society. Active participation in the society's activities, including presenting at meetings, serving on committees, and contributing to the mission of the society, is essential. My first role in the American Society of Breast Surgeons was Program Chair of the 2013 meeting. This allowed me an incredible opportunity to build strong professional relationships within the society. However, that role is an appointed position, and very few will be given such a leadership opportunity initially. For women who aspire to society leadership, I believe that a willingness to serve in multiple roles is critical. Surgical societies are dependent on volunteer service by their members to thrive. One of the best ways to get involved is to volunteer. Many societies have "open calls" for committee positions, contributions to publications or research initiatives, or mentorship roles. My advice is to find a few of those roles that you are passionate about and volunteer to serve. If you are not selected the first time, volunteer again. Be persistent. One of the best ways to get involved in society activities is to make the current leadership aware of how willing you are to participate.

Once you are offered a society role, there are some key steps that can lead to executive leadership. Active engagement is critical. As Stephen Hawking said, "Half the battle is showing up!" I have served on many committees in multiple surgical societies, and many, if not all, of the opportunities I have been given were simply because I was on the conference call or at the meeting and showed up to participate. It is always surprising to me that so many people are given the opportunity to serve on a committee and fail to even show up. Demonstrating leadership qualities by taking the initiative on projects and guiding the group will result in you gaining recognition and ultimately advancing within the society. For instance, I was asked to participate in a consensus panel for our society early in my career. It was intimidating because the group was made up of many of my breast surgeon idols who had far more experience and clout than I did. However, on the first organizing call, I volunteered to write the document and assimilate the group's recommendations. Importantly, I followed through and did it within the deadline outlined by the group. All of those well-known surgeons suddenly knew me and that I delivered on my promise.

I now realize that one of the most important lessons I learned during my many roles in the society prior to becoming president was that I was able to develop my own visionary leadership for the society and its mission. The American Society of Breast Surgeons' mission is to advocate for surgeons who seek excellence in the care of breast patients. This was critical for me to understand as I started my presidency because all of my prior service roles in the society were very task-oriented and designed to deliver information about new advances for patient outcomes. What I was being asked to do as president was quite different. It required a much broader view, ensuring that the members' dues were being used for purposes that would benefit their clinical practices and professional development. That was a bit daunting at first. However, I quickly remembered that I did not need to make decisions in a vacuum. I had many mentors within the society who could provide guidance and support. The specific challenges and obstacles that a society president will face during their tenure vary, but the methods of conflict resolution and overcoming hurdles fortunately do not need to be reinvented year after year. I can now truly say that the most difficult decisions of that year resulted in the most personal satisfaction simply because I was able to learn invaluable lessons that have strengthened my leadership style. I firmly believe that a society president is solely responsible for creating a cohesive and motivated team to drive the society's mission forward, but that requires absolute integrity, empathy, and dedication to do so.

The pathway to becoming the president of a surgical society as a woman is marked by both hurdles and victories. Despite the ongoing challenges related to bias and work-life balance, women surgeons make excellent leaders with distinct and transformative styles. Each president will have a unique story of how they reached that goal, but the underlying foundation of service and volunteerism will be a constant. As more women assume leadership positions, the landscape of surgical societies will continue to evolve, fostering greater inclusivity and innovation. Don't be afraid to reach out to a current or former society president and get their insight on what steps may help you in achieving the same goal. One of the most rewarding aspects of being a society president is the ability to shape the next generation of surgeons who will influence future surgical breakthroughs and societal advancements. That enduring legacy brings great joy.

References

1. Kass RB, Souba WW, Thorndyke LE. Challenges confronting female surgical leaders: Overcoming the barriers. J Surg Res. 2006;132(2):179–187.
2. Troppmann KM, Palis BE, Goodnight JE, et al. Women surgeons in the new millennium. Arch Surg. 2009;144(7):635–642.
3. Greenup RA, Pitt SC. Women in academic surgery: A double-edged scalpel. Acad Med. 2020;95(10):1483–1484.
4. Association of American Medical Colleges. Number and percentage of active physicians by sex and specialty, 2022. Physician Specialty Data Report. https://www.aamc.org/data-reports/workforce/interactive-data/active-physicians-sex-and-specialty-2022. Accessed January 31, 2025.
5. American Society of Breast Surgeons. Past Presidents. https://www.breastsurgeons.org/about/leadership/past_presidents. Accessed January 31, 2025.
6. The American Association for Thoracic Surgery. Past Presidents. https://aats.org/about-the-aats/governance/aats-past-presidents. Accessed January 31, 2025.
7. Southern Surgical Association. Past Presidents. https://web.cvent.com/event/ba9196ae-ccde-4b20-8209-c542a3a2d820/summary. Accessed January 31, 2025.
8. American Academy of Orthopaedic Surgeons. https://aaos.org/about/meet-aaos/leadership-governance/board-of-directors/aaos-presidents-1932-present/. Accessed January 31, 2025.

Chapter 32
Becoming a Chair

Corinne Wee and Marie Crandall

Introduction

Women have made great strides in the medical field, with equal numbers of women and men now matriculating to medical school. This is incredible progress when compared to just 30 years ago, when women made up less than 25% of medical students [1]. Nevertheless, significant disparities remain, especially in academic medicine. Of academic physicians, only 38% are female, and the numbers fall dramatically as rank progresses [2]. Women hold only a small percentage of leadership roles, making up 7% of surgery department chairs [3].

While women face distinct challenges as they ascend to leadership, it is a journey that is both worthwhile and rewarding. This chapter will elaborate on the different strategies in this journey to achieve clinical, academic, and leadership excellence.

C. Wee
Clinical Assistant Professor of Surgery, Division of Plastic and Reconstructive Surgery, Department of Surgery, MetroHealth Medical Center, Cleveland, OH, USA
e-mail: cwee2@metrohealth.org

M. Crandall (✉)
Richard B. Fratianne Professor of Surgery, Case Western Reserve University, Cleveland, OH, USA

Chair of Surgery, MetroHealth, Cleveland, OH, USA
e-mail: mcrandall@metrohealth.org

K. Yoon-Flannery et al. (eds.), *Women in Surgery*,
https://doi.org/10.1007/978-3-032-10971-2_32

Clinical

Exemplifying clinical excellence is essential to being recognized within and outside of one's institution. At every career stage, tracking outcomes on a regular basis is important for self-reflection and continuous improvement. Tracking outcomes can be informal (keeping a personal spreadsheet) or formal (active participation in quality improvement projects). Formal outcomes review can use data-driven assessments such as the American College of Surgeons (ACS) National Surgical Quality Improvement Project (NSQIP), Vizient, and the ACS Trauma Quality Improvement Project (TQIP) to ensure best practices within and beyond one's institution. Different committees dedicated to patient safety exist both on an institutional and national level and provide an opportunity for leadership.

Furthermore, engagement with trainees and advanced practice providers serves as an avenue for both imparting knowledge and gaining new insight. This includes training in the clinical setting as well as participating in journal clubs, didactics, and mentorship.

Active participation in professional societies is also helpful for career growth and gaining recognition. Some groups are specialty-specific (e.g., Society for Surgical Oncology, American Society of Plastic Surgeons) while others may be formed based on identity (e.g., American Medical Women's Association, Society of Black Academic Surgeons). Multispecialty groups such as the American College of Surgeons or the American Medical Association include physicians from multiple specialties and tackle issues such as political or social advocacy, medical training, and academics. All types of groups are important for forming connections. These groups can also provide a resource when encountering clinical or professional challenges. When searching for cause-specific groups or committees, find a mission that you are passionate about and whose cause also bolsters your career goals. Active participation within a group is a great way to shape medicine in a collaborative environment. With experience and time, leadership roles in these groups will also enhance professional standing.

Academic

Providers should seek to advance their fields through scientific inquiry, data collection, and ultimately publishing peer-reviewed articles. Publications and presentations at meetings increase visibility and allow for the sharing of ideas. Meetings are a wonderful place to search for others with similar interests and different perspectives, setting the stage for mentorship, friendship, and/or professional collaboration.

Through presentations and publications, physicians can also increase their academic rank. Physicians generally enter academic practice at either a clinical instructor or assistant professor level and subsequently progress to associate professor, then professor, and then gain tenure. Promotion depends on multiple factors, including research productivity. The mean number of publications to become a full professor of medicine is 20; however, this varies significantly based on specialty and research impact (H-index) [4]. While research is certainly important, higher academic ranks can also be achieved based on grant funding, national/international recognition, leadership roles, and teaching skills. A good candidate for promotion should have a combination of these factors.

Leadership

Leadership roles both within and outside of your institution are important. Institutional committees are important for optimizing processes and quality of care. Selecting committees that complement one's expertise or help develop new skills can be particularly advantageous to both you and your institution. Internal committees often cover topics related to the business of medicine, and improving business literacy is critical to those seeking leadership positions. Familiarity with financial principles such as profit and loss (P&L) statements and earnings before interest, depreciation, and amortization (EBITDA) aids in making informed decisions. Other steps such as obtaining an MBA degree, hiring financial consultants, or developing proficiency in spreadsheets and analysis will enhance one's negotiation skills once in leadership.

In addition to gaining an understanding of business principles, rising leaders should seek opportunities to improve their interpersonal skills through both self-reflection and external sources. "Primal Leadership: Unleashing the Power of Emotional Intelligence [5]," and "Move Fast and Fix Things [6]" are two excellent sources that discuss the importance of emotional intelligence in an evolving workplace. Additionally, participating in courses within and/or outside of your institution can offer valuable insights into leadership skills and strategies.

Media engagement and social media influence can be a double-edged sword, but have become increasingly important in gaining professional recognition. Media presence is another way to boost recognition as a leader, but physicians should be careful not to compromise credibility. The media should be utilized as an opportunity to improve public health and understanding. Social media platforms, when used carefully, can offer a space for academic discourse, advocacy, and policy change.

Challenges Unique to Women

Women may face challenges as they pursue leadership positions; some related to societal culture and others related to biology. Cultural challenges include discrimination, microaggressions, and inherent biases. At every stage of their career, healthcare professionals of all sexes should advocate for a psychologically safe environment. While cultural change takes time, every effort helps to nudge the culture towards a more inclusive one. Acknowledging biases and understanding how to address these helps create a workplace culture where all types of people can succeed.

Even as workplace culture improves, females may encounter challenges that are unique to women. Sometimes referred to as the "motherhood penalty," female physicians who choose to have children face lost productivity when compared to their male counterparts with children. One study showed that female physicians who had children earned 37% less than their male counterparts, compared to only 4% less for those without children [7]. This study looks at the wage gap alone and does not evaluate more subjective losses, such as lost opportunities or delays in promotion.

As all of the steps to leadership require additional time, women generally have less of it. When compared to men, women are nearly twice as likely to have a partner who works full time, spend significantly more time on domestic tasks, and are more likely to face career interruptions related to childcare [8]. Furthermore, women who have reached stages of their career when they are most likely to be considered for leadership roles find themselves in the "sandwich generation"—preoccupied with caring for both children and parents.

When women do overcome these obstacles and obtain leadership positions, this is an achievement to be celebrated. Due to the rarity of female leaders (and especially female leaders of color), this achievement can lead to an overwhelming amount of additional requests—including requests for mentorship, committee positions, and panel placements. These additional requests may contribute to burnout for female chairs, who already hold a demanding position.

Planning Your Pathway

With these strategies in mind, you can begin to plan your pathway to becoming a chair. This pathway begins by obtaining a faculty position within an academic institution. From there, one should work towards leadership roles, advancing from committee leader to a division leader, and eventually vice chair, before advancing to chair. The road does not have to end with becoming a chair! From here, chairwomen can channel their leadership into becoming a dean or seeking an executive leadership position.

As medicine continues to evolve, so do the requirements and strategies to become a chair, and thus, it is necessary to remain current. Annual events, such as "So You Want to Be a Chair," hosted by the Society of Surgical Chairs (SSC) and the ACS Women in Surgery Committee offer helpful and timely advice. As each physician's journey is unique, individual mentorship can be especially valuable to tailor advice to each person's career. Many professional societies, such as the Eastern Association for the Surgery of Trauma (EAST), offer formal mentorship programs which connect senior and junior physicians (EAST Executive Leadership Coaching and Mentoring Program). The Executive Leadership in Academic Medicine (ELAM) program is another wonderful resource for more senior female healthcare professionals; this program has already helped thousands of women achieve their career leadership goals and continues to do so through a part-time fellowship.

Conclusion

My hope with this chapter is to outline a path along which other female physicians can ascend to leadership positions. Deliberate steps towards clinical, academic, and leadership excellence will help pave the way. Once there, we must continue to encourage, guide, and recruit each other along the way. Most importantly, we must remember the challenges before us and work to shape culture and policy to address these.

References

1. Morris, D. B. et al. Diversity of the National Medical Student Body - Four Decades of Inequities. N. Engl. J. Med. 384, 1661–1668 (2021).
2. Richter, K. P. et al. Women Physicians and Promotion in Academic Medicine. N. Engl. J. Med. 383, 2148–2157 (2020).
3. Columbus, A. B. et al. Factors Associated With the Professional Success of Female Surgical Department Chairs: A Qualitative Study. JAMA Surg. 155, 1028–1033 (2020).
4. Zaorsky, N. G. et al. Publication Productivity and Academic Rank in Medicine: A Systematic Review and Meta-Analysis. Acad. Med. 95, 1274–1282 (2020).
5. Goleman, D., Boyatzis, R. & McKee, A. Primal Leadership: Unleashing the Power of Emotional Intelligence.
6. Frei, F. & Morriss, A. Move Fast and Fix Things.
7. Nishida, S., Usui, E., Oshio, T., Masumori, N. & Tsuchihashi, K. Motherhood penalty for female physicians in Japan: evidence from a medical school's alumni data. BMC Health Serv. Res. 24, 1183 (2024).
8. Jolly, S. et al. Gender differences in time spent on parenting and domestic responsibilities by highachieving young physician-researchers. Ann. Intern. Med. 160, 344–353 (2014).

Part VIII
Maintaining Balance and Resilience

Chapter 33
Pregnancy

Kahyun Yoon-Flannery

I am a mother of four children and a breast surgeon in a thriving academic practice. My oldest, the only daughter of ours, was born in my fourth year of medical school—which allowed me to attend all of my general surgery residency interviews fully and visibly pregnant. Keeping up with the work on sub-internships away from home was difficult, but I almost feel like this was a rare opportunity to truly stand out. There still remains a bias against pregnancy in general surgery, although we have made some reasonable progress. I worked my tail off on all of my sub-internships during the height of my first successful pregnancy. I think in a way this did set me apart from the rest of the applicants that the programs were able to see that I was willing to work hard, no matter the circumstances. At the time of residency ranking submission, I received a personal phone call from many programs asking me to rank their program highly.

Achieving four pregnancies during my career was no easy feat. Our first successful pregnancy actually came after a miscarriage and many rounds of a whole lot of injections, medications, and fertility clinic visits. I myself find it so hard to believe that we had to go through it for our only daughter to carry out three additional pregnancies, all with boys, without any assistance (or even planning!).

As I mentor many residents and students, I frequently get asked this particular question: "When is it a good time to have a baby?". My first was during my fourth year of medical school, my second in my PGY 2 year, my third was born a week after my residency graduation, and my fourth was born during my first year in practice. This, I think, would make me an ideal person to perhaps guide anyone to determine the best time to carry out a pregnancy during surgical training. However, every pregnancy at each time presented its own challenges. I definitely would not

K. Yoon-Flannery (✉)
Chief of Women's Cancer Services, Chief of Breast Surgery, Atlanticare Regional Medical Center, Egg Harbor Township, NJ, USA
e-mail: kay.yoonflannery@gmail.com

K. Yoon-Flannery et al. (eds.), *Women in Surgery*,
https://doi.org/10.1007/978-3-032-10971-2_33

recommend anyone to plan to have a baby in PGY 2 year in General Surgery training. Learning how to be a reliable surgical intern is hard enough without a pregnancy, and the second year of General Surgery residency is usually where you really start to learn to operate and learn to conquer others' expectations as well as your own. With a toddler already at home and now an infant, trying to survive my second year of residency that included a trauma surgery rotation at an outside institution was very difficult. There were days that I drove home after spending 30 hours in the trauma ICU and the bay (against ACGME rules, which were bent) just so that I could spend some reasonable time with my daughter, and there were definitely some dangerous moments on the road. In contrast, being pregnant as a chief resident actually was not half bad! I had some control and freedom over my own schedule and the type of cases I was to be a part of (as much control as a surgical residency will allow one to have), although I still remember many attendings asking why I was still coming to do their big cases when I had already matched and I was the size of a mountain. Till the end, I wanted to take advantage of every minute of training. I was not going to run out of my program with people saying, "she's just a breast surgeon".

As a pregnant resident, I was able to arrange all my OB appointments on my post-call days. It did require some advance planning on my part, but staying organized was in my blood as a surgical resident. When I became pregnant as a new attending, however, I found out very fast that there were no more post-call days! Gone were the days when I was able to finally catch up on my medical and dental appointments with some freedom, as long as I stayed up during the day. The patients on my office schedule and the operating room still remained regardless of what happened the evening before during my call week. This created some challenges to allow me to keep up with my OB appointments, and I was not prepared for this. Another challenge I faced as a breast surgeon in practice particularly was dealing with patients with a specific timeline while they were on neoadjuvant systemic therapy. Thankfully, my two wonderful partners not only supported me on this, but they actually were even upset that I was planning on returning to work too soon. I felt, though as someone new in practice, stepping away to recover from a delivery was a luxury I could not afford. In retrospect, I really should have taken the time to heal and recover, but having such supportive partners was a new discovery for me, and I simply did not want to leave my work behind to dump on them.

Now, with my daughter about to start her first year in high school, and the youngest starting first year in elementary school, our household finally is free of all the diapers, breastfeeding, and everything in between. Pregnancies can be so challenging, but parenthood is even more so. My children do not remember the time that I was not present, being on call, sometimes far away from them, but they do now know that mom is here for their football practices and crew sessions. My husband has always been the emergency contact for a variety of in-school and after-school activities, as some aspects of my schedule are not within my own control. Kids are so resilient though. My daughter thinks nothing of calling into the OR to ask me what she thinks is a critical question that needs an answer right away. Mom is always mom first, and the surgeon comes second.

For all of you who are contemplating a pregnancy, my only advice is this: there is no perfect time for a pregnancy, and so any time by default is a good time to become pregnant. Especially if you have a supportive partner who will fill in whatever gaps your career will create.

Chapter 34
Navigating Parenthood and Surgical Careers

Maureen D. Moore

A Dual Identity

I find no other logical way to begin this chapter other than to say—I became pregnant as an intern at an Ivy League institution. It was a time already defined by exhaustion, steep learning curves, and pressure to prove myself. The budding question for me may be why then? Well, to be honest, I didn't really think about it too much. I had friends outside of medicine who were becoming pregnant, and I knew I always wanted to be a mother. My husband and I decided to start a family, and rather quickly that decision was made a reality. I was nervous to tell my program director and my administrative chief resident. Would I be treated differently? Assigned different cases? Thankfully, these questions I had arose after I had become pregnant, so at that juncture, there was not much I could do about it if I was "singled out." Thankfully, I was not. I delivered my baby during the beginning of my second year of residency, in the midst of my transplant rotation—a notoriously demanding service that left little room for rest. Just weeks before delivery, I was unexpectedly diagnosed with listeria, a rare but serious infection requiring a week's hospital stay and a PICC line for antibiotics. Despite this, I went back to work as a pregnant surgical resident 9 days later with my antibiotics and PICC line in tow—come hell or high water, I was going to learn my trade. My program was incredibly supportive with time off and accommodations if needed. At that moment, I realized I had a dual identity—at times one higher on my priority list than the other—I was a mother and a surgeon. My daughter Gracie is the perfect result of my imperfect planning.

M. D. Moore (✉)
Assistant Professor of Surgery, Department of Surgery, Cooper University Hospital, Cooper Medical School of Rowan University, Camden, NJ, USA
e-mail: moore-maureen@cooperhealth.edu

K. Yoon-Flannery et al. (eds.), *Women in Surgery*,
https://doi.org/10.1007/978-3-032-10971-2_34

The Timing Dilemma

When is the "right" time to have children in surgical training/practice? Is it medical school, residency, fellowship, or attending life? In my opinion, as a mother of four children, who has delivered in residency, research, fellowship, and as an attending, there is no perfect time. The myth of the perfect window must be dissolved. Social and professional pressure to delay or "plan perfectly" can lead to other stressors such as difficulty conceiving. The question of when to have children as a woman in surgery can often be framed as a choice between career progression and personal fulfillment. The timing may never feel ideal: medical school may feel too early, residency is too demanding, fellowship is too uncertain, and attending life comes with new pressures to establish oneself and a practice.

Many women wrestle with the fear that pregnancy might be seen as a lack of commitment or a burden to colleagues. Perhaps—like me—you may question if you may be isolated and treated differently. In my experience, it was quite the opposite. My residency program, my fellowship, and my first job as an attending were all supportive of me having children. I was driven by my commitment—my commitment to surgery and my commitment to motherhood. I proved to my colleagues, with the help of great support from my husband and extended family, that I could be a great surgeon and also be a great mother.

Pregnancy in the OR

The demands of long hours on your feet and the physical intensity of operating do not ease with a growing belly. Morning sickness, swelling, and exhaustion that come with pregnancy certainly do not disappear for women surgeons. However, there are subtle ways to help ease the symptoms of pregnancy while navigating surgical residency and practice. For example, since I had morning sickness with all of my pregnancies—my toothbrush and toothpaste were always near me to help with the aftermath. I always knew where the closest bathroom was in case of a sudden need to vomit. I carried small snacks with me in my pocket to help mitigate the feeling of nausea. I wore compression socks to combat the swelling in my legs and never hesitated to put my feet up when I was able. While I was pregnant, I made sure to get to bed as early as I was I could—which meant sacrificing time with my husband and family. Fortunately, my husband and family understood that these sacrifices were for a short 10 months, and my rest was important. With all of this being said, it is important to note that we should not normalize "pushing through" pregnancy when your body is telling you to slow down and rest. As a surgeon and a mother, you have a responsibility to take care of yourself during these strenuous times.

Accommodations and Parental Leave

In 2024, the American Board of Surgery (ABS) put out a revised statement on pregnancy, parental leave, and lactation for practicing surgeons. Below are some bullet points of the revised statement, which can be found on the ABS website:

- "The ACS encourages individualized assessment of requests for reasonable schedule and duty modifications based on pregnancy-related conditions in accordance with applicable federal and state laws."
- "It is appropriate to consider accommodations to call schedule, duty hours, and operative schedule after 30 weeks of pregnancy including cessation of overnight call duties and 24-h call shifts. Pregnant surgeons should be allowed to take short breaks as needed."
- "Pregnant surgeons should avoid exposure to radiation in the operating room. Those in the first trimester of pregnancy should be excused from fluoroscopy cases given the high risk of radiation exposure."
- "The ACS supports parental leave of no less than 6 weeks (vaginal delivery), 8 weeks (cesarean section), and domestic partner leave of not less than 6 weeks."
- "For most individuals, expressing milk for 30–40 min every three to four hours provides sufficient milk for the infant. This accommodation also reduces the risk of developing engorgement, pain, or mastitis. Covered employers are required to provide eligible employees with reasonable breaktime in a private, safe, and convenient place (other than a bathroom) to express breast milk or breastfeed for one year following the birth of a child. These requirements were set forth by the Patient Protection and Affordable Care Act of 2010, which amended Section 7 of the Fair Labor Standards Act.6 Access to a safe, hygienic, and convenient place for the secure storage of expressed milk should also be provided."
- "Individuals should have protected time to express breast milk and have clinic and operating schedule adjustments without bias or penalty."

Accommodations and parental leave have improved certainly since 2014, when I had my first child. With the avocation from many societies including American College of Surgeons (ACS), Association for Women Surgeons (AWS), ACS Resident & Associate Society (RAS), ACS Women in Surgery Committee (WiSC), ACS Young Fellows Association (YFA), the Association of Program Directors in Surgery (APDS), and the Society of Surgical Chairs, these guidelines have permeated through many surgical programs.

Childcare: Logistics, Guilt, and Strategy

I brought home my first child after a 2-day hospital stay. Immediately, I picked up the phone to call the daycare, which assured me my waitlist spot would be available by the time I delivered. On the other end of the phone, I heard, "I am sorry, there is no spot available for your daughter, and a spot will not be open for another two months." Two months? I was due to return to work in 6 weeks—I was fraught with anxiety. My husband, also a full-time employee at his job, was not able to take off work for that long either. Surreptitiously, I was able to secure a nanny who ended up being a true blessing in our lives. My husband, another blessing, stayed with our children every other weekend that I was on call.

With unpredictable hours, long calls, and weekend coverage, the traditional 9 to 5 childcare model rarely fits a surgical schedule. Securing reliable coverage often means piecing together nannies or babysitters, daycare, night shifts, family support, and certainly emergency coverage. Often, the mental load of coordinating it all can be heavier than the clinical workload itself. I am not sure I have resounding advice as to how to deal with the logistics, other than to say surround yourself with a large support system. I had other surgical residents, friends, and family, in addition to my husband's astounding scarifies, to help care for our children.

Beyond logistics lies a deeper emotional toll: the guilt of leaving before your child wakes up or missing milestones while you are scrubbed in the operating room. This guilt can be compounded to perform full capacity at both roles—an unrealistic expectation. As I said in the paragraph above—the dual identity of a surgeon mother can be obtained—but often one takes priority over the other in a shifting fashion. Over time, the management of motherhood and a surgical career can get easier. I have learned to tailor my life to both roles. When I am off from work, I am dedicated to all four of my children. I ensure my time with them is time well spent. As they have grown older, they are now intrigued by my daily schedule and patients. When I come home from work, they ask me about the details of my operations. In school, my kids have proudly proclaimed their mother is a surgeon! All of this is to say, there will be difficulties with logistics that can be overcome with strategies and a support system. As far as the guilt—it will remain—but rest assured, your children are your biggest fans and supporters.

Conclusion: Redefining Success

Navigating parenthood and surgical careers comes with a redefinition of success. Perhaps you started your surgical career with the definition of success as the number of cases performed or as obtaining the role of administrative chief resident. With parenthood, success may mean performing fewer operations in order to be there for your child's school play. Adaptation and flexibility are needed for a dual identity as a surgeon mother. Support systems and strategy are needed to be a successful surgeon mother. Love of both your career and children need not be mutually exclusive—embrace your dual identity.

Chapter 35
Family Planning

Aditi M. Kapil

As a trauma surgeon, who has been fortunate enough to complete my family, I have endured the spectrum of family planning challenges from abortion to IVF to complicated pregnancies during my surgical career.

Surgical training is usually at the peak reproductive time of women's life span, and due to various reasons, including lack of support, bias, discrimination, time limitations, intense work hours, and toxic exposure, many women delay childbearing until after training. This delay has been shown to increase the use of assisted reproductive technologies (ART) by surgeons.

A 2014 study states that 32% women surgeons reported fertility difficulty. In the general population in the USA, 10% of women use ART to attempt pregnancy, in comparison to 76% in the surgical field. The first pregnancy for most female surgeons is at 33 years old, a decade later than the national average of 23. The highest rates of infertility in this 2014 study were ENT, general surgery, and orthopedics.

Most women delay pregnancy due to the demand for surgical residency, lack of support within the program, and bias against pregnancy. A cohort study in 2024 still shows that female residents are likely to delay pregnancies compared to male residents. In comparison with the partners of the male residents, female residents were more likely to experience obstetric complications and postpartum depression. Pregnancy/parenthood mistreatment was shown to be associated with increased burnout and thoughts of attrition. Surprisingly, postpartum depression in both female residents and partners of male residents was shown to be associated with resident burnout. Without increased support for family planning for our surgical residents, gender inequality will increase, and women will continue to delay childbearing to later years.

A. M. Kapil (✉)
Assistant Professor of Surgery, Yale School of Medicine, New Haven, CT, USA
e-mail: aditi.kapil@yale.edu

K. Yoon-Flannery et al. (eds.), *Women in Surgery*,
https://doi.org/10.1007/978-3-032-10971-2_35

The data that has accumulated should allow programs to create support systems for pregnant surgeons starting from the top down. The ability to have children during training would allow women to have children in a safe age range and decrease the need for ART due to age and pregnancy complications. The path of ART for the female surgeon involves the investment of many doctors' appointments and procedures, as well as the emotional toll, which is often not accounted for. Investing in the women surgeons' short period of pregnancy is small to ensure a long career of 20–30 years of talent.

As we want to bring the best candidates to our subspecialties, programs must give space to allow for family planning, which must include both men and women. In my own surgical career, I can see how it has changed where it was openly frowned upon to be a pregnant surgical resident during training to our female residents feeling more comfortable being pregnant during their clinical training. I think this will continue to improve as we continue to shed more light on issues such as family planning, pregnancy, and parenthood.

However, change is slow, and waiting for the perfect opportunity for family planning during surgical training is likely impossible. As someone who waited until after training, I endured the rigors of IVF while I was continuing to practice medicine, with many appointments, procedures, and emotional ups/downs of the process. If family planning is important, I would not allow surgical training to be a barrier. You will never get back the years of your fertility, whereas surgery will be waiting for you when you get back.

References

1. Dason ES, Maxim M, Gesink D, et al. Medical Students' Perspectives on Family Planning and Impact on Specialty Choice. JAMA Surg. 2024;159(2):170–178. doi:https://doi.org/10.1001/jamasurg.2023.6392
2. Li RD, Janczewski LM, Eng JS, Foote DC, Wu C, Johnson JK, Easter SR, Kim E, Buyske J, Turner PL, Nasca TJ, Bilimoria KY, Hu YY, Rangel EL. Pregnancy and Parenthood Among US Surgical Residents. JAMA Surg. 2024 Oct 1;159(10):1127-1137. doi: https://doi.org/10.1001/jamasurg.2024.2399. PMID: 39018050; PMCID: PMC11255977.
3. Patel A, Wilson CA, Davidson J, Lam JY, Graham ME, Seemann NM. The Intersection of Family Planning and Perception of Career Advancement in General Surgery. J Surg Res. 2024 Apr;296:481-488. doi: https://doi.org/10.1016/j.jss.2024.01.017. Epub 2024 Feb 6. PMID: 38325010.
4. Phillips EA, Nimeh T, Braga J, Lerner LB. Does a surgical career affect a woman's childbearing and fertility? A report on pregnancy and fertility trends among female surgeons. J Am Coll Surg. 2014 Nov;219(5):944-50. doi: https://doi.org/10.1016/j.jamcollsurg.2014.07.936. Epub 2014 Aug 1. PMID: 25260684.
5. Rangel EL, Castillo-Angeles M, Easter SR, et al. Incidence of Infertility and Pregnancy Complications in US Female Surgeons. JAMA Surg. 2021;156(10):905–915. doi:https://doi.org/10.1001/jamasurg.2021.3301
6. Stefanou AJ. Fertility and Pregnancy: How Do These Affect Family Planning and Surgeon Health? Clin Colon Rectal Surg. 2023 Mar 8;36(5):327-332. doi: https://doi.org/10.1055/s-0043-1764240. PMID: 37564346; PMCID: PMC10411105.

7. Yau A, Lentskevich MA, Ahmed KS, Rangel EL, Gosain AK. Female Surgeons and Physicians Experience Greater Infertility Rates and Pregnancy Complications Than Other Professional Women. Am Surg. 2024 Apr;90(4):494-501. doi: https://doi.org/10.1177/00031348231216489. Epub 2023 Nov 17. PMID: 37975740.

Chapter 36
Support Systems for Surgeon Parents

Alexis Colley and Julie Ann Sosa

Introduction

Surgical training is lengthy and overlaps with the most common childbearing years. Increasing numbers of residents are starting families during this time period, yet many may still delay family building, leave surgical training, or choose specialties they deem more family-friendly [12, 14]. Those who do bear children during training face higher rates of infertility, pregnancy loss, and major pregnancy complications [10]. The challenges of parenthood as a resident are coupled with stigma (perceived and actual), as well as multiple layers (e.g., logistical, physical, emotional, and financial) of stress that further compound the impacts of rigorous surgical training [9]. Despite these challenges, residents who become parents are resilient, and data show no differences in caseload, attrition, or exam passage rates between female surgical residents who have been pregnant when compared with other residents [15].

Prior research has shown that negative perceptions about pregnancy and childrearing exist among surgical trainees. For example, among female surgeons, 73% say they have witnessed colleagues make negative comments about pregnant residents or childbearing during training [11]. This stigma affects women more than men, with 61% of female surgical trainees (compared to 16% of their male peers)

A. Colley
Department of Surgery, University of California San Francisco (UCSF),
San Francisco, CA, USA
e-mail: alexis.colley@ucsf.edu

J. A. Sosa (✉)
Leon Goldman, MD Distinguished Professor of Surgery and Chair, Department of Surgery,
Professor, Department of Medicine, Affiliated Faculty, Philip R. Lee Institute for Health
Policy Studies, University of California San Francisco (UCSF), San Francisco, CA, USA
e-mail: julie.sosa@ucsf.edu

K. Yoon-Flannery et al. (eds.), *Women in Surgery*,
https://doi.org/10.1007/978-3-032-10971-2_36

believing that they would be viewed unfavorably if they had a child during residency, and 82% of women (60% of men) believing childbearing would adversely impact their career [8]. These beliefs are also pervasive among some surgical leaders; 61% of residency program directors reported that becoming a parent negatively affects female trainees' work, and 32% perceived that female trainees who are mothers had lower levels of well-being compared to their male counterparts who are fathers [12]. Stigma around childbearing may impact trainees' willingness to advocate for themselves [11] and may make them even more vulnerable to the already higher risk for pregnancy-related complications [10].

Experiences of family building during surgical training clearly impact current trainees; for example, up to 40% of women who have children during residency have strongly considered leaving the specialty. They also affect future generations of potential surgeons, in that 30% of the same cohort would advise female medical students against pursuing a surgical career [11]. Institutions should work to understand and eliminate stigma associated with choices made in the personal realm; the decision to have children during residency is just such a decision. To do so, accurate and relevant information about policies pertaining to family leave must be made easily accessible to prospective and current trainees. Residency program leadership should devise structures of support for those in their charge (e.g., lactation and family leave policies) and educate faculty on the expected needs for various stages of family planning; essential information includes the need for time away for prenatal visits and periodic breaks from the operating room to administer medications or to express milk [5].

While all segments of the parenting journey carry unique challenges, the period of time after returning to work from parental leave is known to be among the most difficult [13].

> This was true for me (A.C.) when I returned to work after having my first daughter mid-way through my third year of general surgery residency training. Upon my return, I found my days overwhelming and discouraging. The excitement and hope of pregnancy had been replaced with an invisible burden of added caregiving responsibilities for my child on top of the busy clinical schedule I had. Between severe sleep deprivation, physical recovery from pregnancy, and lactation needs, this was the most challenging period of my life. An even greater burden, however, was the profound emotional toll of being away from my new baby. Despite what seemed at times insurmountable, I was fortunate to have several strong, caring, and vocal mentors who provided logistical insights and a sense of community. I received advice and messages of solidarity from several of the female faculty with children, including things like "always pump on the way to work" and "email your attendings ahead of time [to let them know about your needs during cases]". Though helpful, the content of their messages was not as impactful to me as knowing that they represented a community of moms who had been through similar experiences and had emerged as excellent surgeons, caring mentors, and dedicated mothers. With time, I began to find a way to integrate my new life with my resident life and continue working on this today. I sought to make the type of mentorship I had (as well as that which I had lacked) available for others who are also planning on raising families.

This served as an important part of the inspiration for the UCSF Parenting in Surgery Initiative.

The Parenting in Surgery Initiative is a comprehensive program available to all surgical trainees in our Department of Surgery, as well as a modality to provide information on best practices to trainee parents at other institutions. The initiative was designed to provide information and education and normalize family-building with a particular emphasis on the challenges unique to surgeons (Fig. 36.1). The program was launched in August 2023 with enthusiastic backing of the department's leadership, including the Chair of Surgery (JAS), the general, plastic, and vascular surgery residency program directors, the Director of Gender Equity, and the Muriel Steele Society (a community of surgeons focused on development and support for surgeons who are women and other gender minorities).

The Parenting in Surgery Initiative includes the following:

- *Guidelines on Family Leave*—Despite the American Board of Surgery (ABS) publicizing its policies that apply to having children during training, only 4% of surgical residents were aware of the policies [1], and only 6% of programs had information about leave policies on their websites [3]. The Parenting in Surgery Initiative resources (available publicly on the program's website at https://surgeryresidentportal.ucsf.edu/policies/family-planning/parenting-in-surgery.aspx) summarize the ABS policy on Family Leave for Surgical Trainees for residency and fellowship to help residents plan for family leave time. A member of our educational staff also meets with all trainees planning for family leave to help them understand the amount of time available for leave according to both the

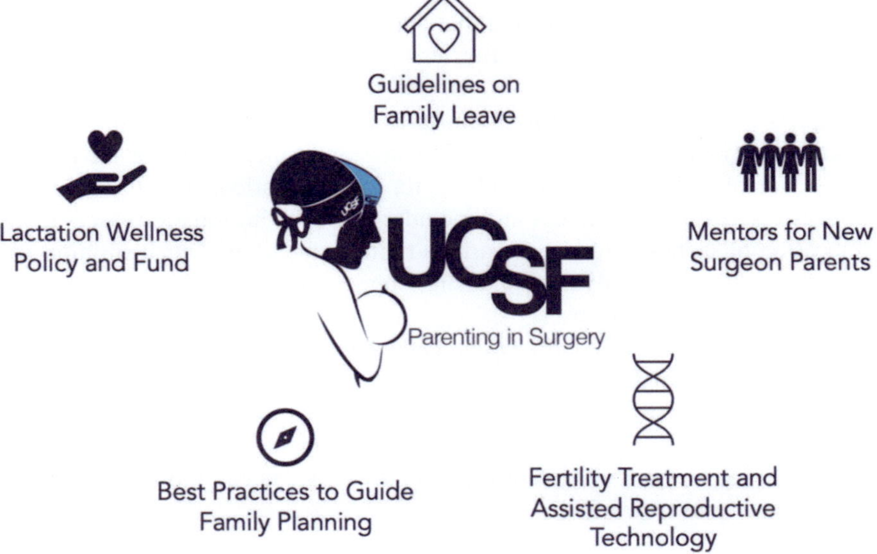

Fig. 36.1 The five components of the Parenting in Surgery initiative are designed to robustly support childbearing and childrearing during surgical training

Accreditation Council for Graduate Medical Education and ABS, integrate scheduling preferences, and connect them with human resources.

- *Mentors for New Surgeon Parents*—Mentorship has been shown to contribute positively to both career development and retention for surgeons, yet two-thirds of pregnant residents found mentorship for integrating a surgical career with family to be lacking [7]. In our Parenting in Surgery program, residents and faculty are matched one-on-one for an additional layer of support. To solicit mentors, emails are sent to individuals who are known by program leadership to have children. Mentors self-identify as being willing to be paired with a trainee for a minimum of three meetings. New parent trainees select a compatible mentor from a list of volunteers and are introduced by a faculty liaison. Notably, mentors are of all genders, and trainees can choose to be paired with a mentor that suits their needs (e.g., based on gender, specialty, or other characteristic).
- *Best Practices to Guide Family Planning*—Our Parenting in Surgery Initiative resource provides practical guidance on expected challenges facing the pregnant surgeon, from preconception to postpartum recovery and return to work. The document outlines the responsibilities of the resident and training program at each stage and carries with it the expectation that faculty and trainees will be familiar with the policies (Table 36.1).
- *Lactation Wellness Policy and Fund*—One of the main challenges for new mothers returning to work is lactation wellness and breastfeeding. Among 246 female surgical residents who gave birth during residency, 67% indicated that they did not have adequate time for pumping, and 56% rarely had access to a lactation room, with 64% saying that these factors contributed to a shortened duration of breastfeeding [4]. Barriers to support for lactating trainees, as identified by program directors, include residents' discomfort in making a request to leave the operating room to express milk, as well as poor understanding by faculty of the practical logistics and time needed for the process [2]. Our resource outlines guidelines for lactation-oriented wellness among faculty and surgical trainees and includes practical information, such as the location of lactation rooms at various training facilities. Our institution has also committed to providing financial support (up to $500) for trainees to cover lactation supply costs.
- *Fertility Treatment and Assisted Reproductive Technology*—Due to the pressures of residency, many female surgeons delay childbirth and are more likely to need assisted reproductive technology (ART) [5]. The Parenting in Surgery Initiative includes a summary of information about ART and a list of faculty members at our institution who have volunteered to provide mentorship to residents interested in, or pursuing, ART.

Table 36.1 Best practices to guide family planning

Time period	Anticipated challenges	Trainee responsibilities	Program responsibilities
Preconception	Time required to attend medical appointments Physical and emotional changes associated with hormone administration for fertility	Communicate with residency program director (PD) about time needed for appointments and/or to administer medications	Keep resident endeavors around fertility confidential Accommodate the resident's needs for fertility and family planning Provide residents with the option to reduce or eliminate the 24-h call/night float that can adversely affect cycles
First trimester	Nausea and fatigue Limit fluoroscopy exposure (throughout pregnancy) and toxic exposure (heated intraperitoneal chemotherapy (HIPEC), sevoflurane) Higher risk of miscarriage than in other trimesters	Notify PD of pregnancy (either in the first or second trimester) If desired, meet with PD to discuss reducing 24-h shifts and night float Consider dosimeter badge(s) to monitor radiation exposure Notify rotation director and/or PD for contingency planning regarding toxic exposure	Designated PD meets with trainee and provides parenthood support packet Make accommodation within the schedule to allow for the desired parental leave Postpone rotations that have prolonged radiation exposure (i.e., vascular surgery) If requested, work with residents to reduce or eliminate 24-h shifts and night float
Second trimester	Obstetrics appointments Prenatal workup (anatomy, prenatal ultrasound, amniocentesis, chorionic villus sampling, etc.)	Communicate with team members (co-residents, APPs, and faculty) time that is needed for appointments and testing Select mentor	Prepare paperwork for parental leave 2–3 months before Check in with mentor (at least three times during pregnancy/postpartum period) Check in with a designated member of education leadership (during each phase of pregnancy and monthly if needed)
Third trimester	Antenatal testing Physical limitations of mobility and risk of preterm labor	Work with faculty to allow for breaks during long cases (for patient and trainee safety)	List of recommended rotations
Parental leave	Guidelines on family leave for surgical trainees		Program arranges for call coverage during leave and requires no "make-up" call from the resident on leave

(continued)

Table 36.1 (continued)

Time period	Anticipated challenges	Trainee responsibilities	Program responsibilities
Postpartum period	Refer to Lactation Wellness Policy Physical changes associated with the postpartum period Emotional challenges with returning to work and being away from the child	Be familiar with the lactation policy Connect with a lactation champion at each site Close communication with team members, including attendings, if any intra-operative accommodations are anticipated	Consider transition rotation Continue check-ins with "Surgeon New Parent" mentor Continue check-in with the designated member of education leadership: check on the trainee's emotional transition back to work The designated program point person will contact rotation directors and faculty to make them aware of the need for protected time for pumping, as outlined in the Lactation Wellness Policy

Conclusion

Increasing numbers of Americans, particularly women, are caring for both their own children and aging family members, yet this work is often unacknowledged and lacking support from employers [6]. Similarly, surgical residents who become parents during their training face numerous challenges, including logistical, emotional, financial, and societal pressures. There is still a perception of a stigma that is associated with balancing parenthood and professional development. To address these issues and promote inclusivity, UCSF Surgery has launched the Parenting in Surgery Initiative, a comprehensive program designed to support trainees who are planning for—and/or raising—families. This initiative includes resources such as family leave guidelines, mentorship programs, lactation support, and information on fertility treatments, all aimed at normalizing family building and reducing stigma in surgical training. By fostering a supportive community and implementing practical policies, we hope to empower surgeon-parents while enhancing recruitment and retention of a diverse surgical workforce.

Disclosures JAS is a member of the Data Monitoring Committee of the Medullary Thyroid Cancer Consortium Registry supported by Novo Nordisk, Astra Zeneca, and Eli Lilly. Institutional research funding was received from Exelixis and Eli Lilly.

References

1. Altieri, M. S., Salles, A., Bevilacqua, L. A., Brunt, L. M., Mellinger, J. D., Gooch, J. C., & Pryor, A. D. (2019). Perceptions of Surgery Residents About Parental Leave During Training. *JAMA Surg, 154*(10), 952-958. https://doi.org/10.1001/jamasurg.2019.2985

2. Castillo-Angeles, M., Smink, D. S., & Rangel, E. L. (2021). Perspectives of US General Surgery Program Directors on Cultural and Fiscal Barriers to Maternity Leave and Postpartum Support During Surgical Training. *JAMA Surg*, *156*(7), 647-653. https://doi.org/10.1001/jamasurg.2021.1807

3. Engelbrecht-Wiggans, E. A., Sundel, M. H., Newland, J. J., Seyoum, N., & Brown, R. F. (2024). Parental leave policies in general surgery residencies. *Am J Surg*, *233*, 25-28. https://doi.org/10.1016/j.amjsurg.2023.12.017

4. Golestani, S., Cardenas, T., Koepp, K., Efird, J., Teixeira, P. G., Mery, M., Dubose, J., Trust, M. D., Bach, M., Ali, S., & Brown, C. V. R. (2024). Barriers to Breastfeeding During Surgery Residency. *J Surg Educ*, *81*(4), 551-555. https://doi.org/10.1016/j.jsurg.2023.12.017

5. Knell, J., Kim, E. S., & Rangel, E. L. (2023). The Challenges of Parenthood for Female Surgeons: The Current Landscape and Future Directions. *J Surg Res*, *288*, A1-A8. https://doi.org/10.1016/j.jss.2023.02.042

6. Lei, L., Leggett, A. N., & Maust, D. T. (2023). A national profile of sandwich generation caregivers providing care to both older adults and children. *J Am Geriatr Soc*, *71*(3), 799-809. https://doi.org/10.1111/jgs.18138

7. Moore, A. L., Smink, D. S., & Rangel, E. L. (2022). A Pregnant Pause-Time to Address Mentorship for Expectant Residents. *JAMA Surg*. https://doi.org/10.1001/jamasurg.2022.1835

8. Pham, D. T., Stephens, E. H., Antonoff, M. B., Colson, Y. L., Dildy, G. A., Gaur, P., Correa, A. M., Litle, V. R., & Blackmon, S. H. (2014). Birth trends and factors affecting childbearing among thoracic surgeons. *Ann Thorac Surg*, *98*(3), 890-895. https://doi.org/10.1016/j.athoracsur.2014.05.041

9. Rangel, E. L., Castillo-Angeles, M., Changala, M., Haider, A. H., Doherty, G. M., & Smink, D. S. (2018). Perspectives of pregnancy and motherhood among general surgery residents: A qualitative analysis. *Am J Surg*, *216*(4), 754-759. https://doi.org/10.1016/j.amjsurg.2018.07.036

10. Rangel, E. L., Castillo-Angeles, M., Easter, S. R., Atkinson, R. B., Gosain, A., Hu, Y. Y., Cooper, Z., Dey, T., & Kim, E. (2021). Incidence of Infertility and Pregnancy Complications in US Female Surgeons. *JAMA Surg*, *156*(10), 905-915. https://doi.org/10.1001/jamasurg.2021.3301

11. Rangel, E. L., Smink, D. S., Castillo-Angeles, M., Kwakye, G., Changala, M., Haider, A. H., & Doherty, G. M. (2018). Pregnancy and Motherhood During Surgical Training. *JAMA Surg*, *153*(7), 644-652. https://doi.org/10.1001/jamasurg.2018.0153

12. Sandler, B. J., Tackett, J. J., Longo, W. E., & Yoo, P. S. (2016). Pregnancy and Parenthood among Surgery Residents: Results of the First Nationwide Survey of General Surgery Residency Program Directors. *J Am Coll Surg*, *222*(6), 1090-1096. https://doi.org/10.1016/j.jamcollsurg.2015.12.004

13. Shifflette, V., Hambright, S., Amos, J. D., Dunn, E., & Allo, M. (2018). The pregnant female surgical resident. *Adv Med Educ Pract*, *9*, 365-369. https://doi.org/10.2147/AMEP.S140738

14. Smith, C., Galante, J. M., Pierce, J. L., & Scherer, L. A. (2013). The surgical residency baby boom: changing patterns of childbearing during residency over a 30-year span. *J Grad Med Educ*, *5*(4), 625-629. https://doi.org/10.4300/JGME-D-12-00334.1

15. Todd, A. R., Cawthorn, T. R., & Temple-Oberle, C. (2020). Pregnancy and Parenthood Remain Challenging During Surgical Residency: A Systematic Review. *Acad Med*, *95*(10), 1607-1615. https://doi.org/10.1097/ACM.0000000000003351

Chapter 37
Side Gigs

Kahyun Yoon-Flannery

I am an avid cruiser. As we are a family of six, especially when the kids were in their toddler ages, it was hard to choose a vacation where we as parents would actually be able to enjoy our time as well as the kids. Disney cruises, while costly, gave us many avenues as a family to achieve this common goal. The kids' club was insanely beautiful and fun, where every day the kids would ask to be dropped off for hours, while the adults-only section provided much-needed respite for my husband and me. Because I had no knowledge of Disney cruises or cruises in general when we started, we used a travel agent. She came to us without an additional cost, and her commission from Disney directly would allow her to help us book the appropriate trip arrangements. We probably used the same agent no fewer than 5 times—on different sailings on different ships, sometimes even with friends or family. And with each trip, I was actually giving more feedback to my agent as to what worked best compared to what she had provided us. One night, it dawned on me. How hard could it be to become a Disney travel agent? If I put myself through a surgical residency with four kids in tow, surely this could not be that difficult. I enrolled in an online course through Disney to receive various forms of training on all Disney-related vacations. I would listen to the sessions on my laptop in bed, where my husband would just quietly watch me and say, "Is this something you really need to do?" and sigh and go back to sleep.

After countless hours of training sessions that were really not difficult at all and actually a lot of fun, and filing for various forms for tax purposes, I created my own travel agency. My sole purpose in creating this originally was to retain my own information from my own trips! Why should I use an agent and allow her to collect commission when I was the one providing much information? This led to booking so many trips, not only personal but also for those of friends and family.

K. Yoon-Flannery (✉)
Chief of Women's Cancer Services, Chief of Breast Surgery, Atlanticare Regional Medical Center, Egg Harbor Township, NJ, USA
e-mail: kay.yoonflannery@gmail.com

K. Yoon-Flannery et al. (eds.), *Women in Surgery*,
https://doi.org/10.1007/978-3-032-10971-2_37

205

This opportunity opened my eyes. I knew so many folks in medicine looked for alternatives to their clinical practice and were wildly successful. There are so many courses on this, actually, through a number of resources. I never thought I would bring myself to do anything other than my day job as a breast surgeon. However, once my "career" as a Disney travel agent took off, I suddenly was able to find additional opportunities, including physician consulting, providing input to a variety of medical device companies. I decided from the beginning that I would only choose projects or companies that would allow me to (1) provide my honest feedback and (2) contribute to medicine in some meaningful way. I happened to use a product during my cases that allowed me to perform a clinical study that led to a significant finding in my field. Suddenly speaking on behalf of a medical company became very easy, as all I was doing was describing how I was able to transform my own practice using a particular product. The speaking engagements were actually not stressful and gave me feedback as to how best to utilize this product to transform breast surgery practice. In doing so, I was able to create a limited liability company (LLC) that also allowed me to utilize tax advantages that were not available to me as an employed surgeon. As a physician in a consulting LLC, there are several ways to consider tax advantages as long as they are related to my consulting activities, and there are many resources focusing on this nowadays. Believe it or not, being able to do this also allowed me to travel more and interact more openly with others in my field, but it also opened many networking opportunities that would allow me to grow outside of my comfort zone.

I have known a number of physicians who have transitioned fully from their clinical practice to what used to be their alternate career paths. As rates of burnout become so devastatingly significant in the field of medicine, side gigs can offer an additional way to look beyond everyday life in medicine, not only by offering additional sources of income, but more in the ways of creativity. Whether it is physician consulting, travel agency, or property rentals, our ability to stay organized and deliberate in our decisions can certainly afford us with means to further our life goals.

Chapter 38
Strategies for Mental Health and Wellness in Female Surgeons

Ashwini Paranjpe and Kandace P. McGuire

The Burden and Culture of Stoicism in Surgery

In addition to these cultural expectations, the surgical training environment itself can reinforce unhealthy coping mechanisms. Long hours, hierarchical structures, and a lack of structured wellness education may lead trainees to adopt maladaptive behaviors early in their careers. Female surgeons often feel pressure to outperform peers to gain credibility, compounding stress levels and reinforcing the internalization of mental distress. Promoting open dialogue about mental health during training could normalize vulnerability and reduce stigma across all levels of surgical education.

Surgical culture has long valued stoicism, grit, and detachment—traits that have enabled surgeons to navigate complex cases and high-pressure environments. However, this same culture can discourage vulnerability, emotional expression, and help-seeking behaviors. Studies have shown that surgeons face high rates of burnout, depression, and even suicidal ideation, with female surgeons at greater risk due to additional systemic and societal stressors [6, 11].

Female surgeons often encounter discrimination, pay inequity, lack of mentorship, and work-life imbalance at higher rates than their male counterparts [2]. These disparities compound the psychological toll of surgical practice, making the development and integration of wellness strategies critical for this population.

A. Paranjpe (✉)
Breast Surgical Oncology, Department of Surgery, Virginia Commonwealth University, Richmond, VA, USA
e-mail: ashwini.paranjpe@vcuhealth.org

K. P. McGuire
Chief of Breast Surgery, Professor of Surgery, Department of Surgery, Virginia Commonwealth University, Richmond, VA, USA
e-mail: kandace.mcguire@vcuhealth.org

K. Yoon-Flannery et al. (eds.), *Women in Surgery*,
https://doi.org/10.1007/978-3-032-10971-2_38

Moreover, emotional wellness strategies should be proactively integrated into institutional frameworks. Scheduled mental health check-ins, the availability of trauma-informed counselors, and formal mentorship programs can all serve as preventive tools. The creation of reflective writing programs and Schwartz Rounds is an additional structured approach proven to facilitate healing conversations among healthcare professionals. These interventions can create safe spaces for surgeons to discuss emotional experiences and derive collective support.

Emotional Wellness: Processing the Workload

Another often-overlooked physical wellness factor is sleep. Surgeons frequently experience chronic sleep deprivation, which has been linked to impaired cognitive function, reduced emotional regulation, and increased risk of medical errors. Institutions should explore the impact of flexible scheduling, shift limits, and fatigue risk management strategies to protect surgeons' ability to rest and recover adequately.

Emotional wellness encompasses the ability to recognize, understand, and manage emotions in healthy ways. For surgeons, emotional processing is often deferred or suppressed in the interest of clinical detachment and professional decorum. Yet, evidence suggests that reflective practices such as journaling, peer debriefing, or structured support groups can help process adverse events, reduce moral distress, and foster emotional resilience [7].

The concept of "second victim" syndrome, wherein clinicians experience trauma after an adverse patient outcome, is particularly relevant to surgeons. Female surgeons may feel intensified guilt or self-doubt due to societal expectations around empathy and perfectionism [10]. Establishing institutional norms for emotional debriefing and peer support can help normalize emotional recovery as part of surgical professionalism.

Institutional investment in affinity groups and networking events can provide critical relational infrastructure for women in surgery. Additionally, mentoring networks such as peer-to-peer or multilevel mentoring can help prevent isolation. For academic surgeons, participation in national specialty organizations and attending women-in-medicine leadership retreats has shown benefits in reinforcing identity, building community, and preventing burnout.

Physical Health as a Foundation for Mental Wellness

Residency programs could consider incorporating formal financial education into their curricula to mitigate long-term financial stress. Topics might include understanding contracts, debt management, negotiating salaries, and retirement planning. Female surgeons may especially benefit from coaching on navigating financial negotiations and advocating for equitable compensation structures. A financially secure surgeon is less burdened by external stress and more likely to make values-aligned career decisions.

While surgical work is physically demanding, it is not inherently health-promoting. Long hours, irregular sleep, and high stress levels often lead to musculoskeletal issues, chronic fatigue, and poor cardiovascular health [12]. Furthermore, surgeons may neglect their own health needs while prioritizing patients.

Regular physical activity is strongly linked to reduced symptoms of depression and anxiety, improved sleep quality, and enhanced cognitive performance [9]. For female surgeons, integrating brief but consistent forms of movement—such as yoga, walking meetings, or stretching routines—can provide tangible physical and psychological benefits. Access to protected time and institutional wellness programs further supports this integration.

Integrating mindfulness into daily routines need not be time-intensive. Even 5–10 min guided meditations before or after cases can make a substantial impact on focus and stress reduction. Mobile apps, such as Headspace or Insight Timer, can provide accessible tools. For those who identify with a spiritual tradition, reengagement with community worship or contemplative practices may serve as a grounding and rejuvenating ritual amidst professional demands.

Social Connection and Community Support

Data transparency regarding gender equity, wellness program outcomes, and promotion rates can hold institutions accountable and guide continuous improvement. Furthermore, wellness should be included as a metric in faculty evaluations and department quality dashboards. Incorporating mental health leave policies and crisis intervention services ensures that well-being is prioritized not just rhetorically, but operationally.

Despite frequent interaction with patients and colleagues, many surgeons experience professional isolation. This paradox is particularly pronounced among women in surgery, who may be underrepresented in their departments or excluded from informal networking opportunities [1].

Strong social connections are a protective factor against burnout and emotional distress. Female surgeons benefit from both intra-professional communities—such as the Association of Women Surgeons—and broader social networks that extend beyond medicine. Participation in nonmedical hobbies, family activities, or local volunteerism can restore a sense of identity and purpose beyond the operating room.

Financial Literacy and Psychological Safety

Financial stress is another underrecognized contributor to poor mental health among physicians. Female surgeons, in particular, may experience unique financial challenges due to gender pay gaps, delayed earnings from prolonged training, and a lack of early financial education. The term "HENRY" (High Earner, Not Rich Yet) captures the phenomenon of physicians with high incomes but limited net worth due to debt and lifestyle inflation.

Improving financial literacy, consulting with fiduciary advisors, and learning about debt management and investment strategies can reduce anxiety and increase long-term autonomy [5]. Institutions should offer workshops or mentorship focused on financial wellness as part of broader professional development.

Mindfulness, Spirituality, and Purpose

Mindfulness-based practices have been shown to reduce burnout, increase empathy, and improve well-being among physicians [3]. These practices include meditation, breathwork, guided reflection, and cognitive reframing. For some surgeons, spirituality or a connection to a greater purpose—whether religious or philosophical—provides a sense of grounding and meaning in the face of loss, uncertainty, and high expectations.

The Japanese concept of "Ikigai," which translates roughly to "reason for being," aligns with many surgeons' desire to serve, grow, and contribute. Identifying and nurturing this personal sense of purpose can enhance emotional endurance and career satisfaction [4].

Institutional Responsibility and Cultural Change

While individual strategies are essential, lasting impact requires systemic change. Organizations must take responsibility for fostering psychological safety, promoting gender equity, and normalizing wellness. Programs that include confidential mental health access, protected time for self-care, transparent promotion criteria, and mentorship for underrepresented groups have been shown to reduce burnout and improve retention [8].

Leadership buy-in is critical. Female surgeons in leadership roles should advocate for structural changes that support wellness—not as a luxury, but as a prerequisite for high-quality, sustainable care.

Conclusion

Mental health and wellness are essential to the longevity and success of female surgeons. By addressing emotional, physical, social, financial, and spiritual well-being through evidence-based strategies and systemic reform, the surgical community can foster a more inclusive, supportive, and resilient environment. The path to well-being is not linear, but it must be intentional—and shared (Appendix A).

Appendix A Evidence-Based Wellness Strategies

Strategy	Description	Evidence source
Mindfulness meditation	Regular mindfulness practice to reduce anxiety, increase emotional regulation.	Fortney et al. [3]
Peer support groups	Structured discussions with colleagues to debrief emotionally taxing cases.	Scott et al. [10]
Physical exercise	Moderate aerobic exercise 3x/week to improve mood and sleep.	Rebar et al. [9]
Financial coaching	Workshops on debt management, salary negotiation, and investment.	Grischkan et al. [5]

References

1. Chambers, C. C., Ihnow, S. B., Monroe, E. J., & Suleiman, L. I. (2018). Women in orthopaedic surgery: Population trends in trainees and practicing surgeons. The Journal of Bone and Joint Surgery, 100(17), e116. https://doi.org/10.2106/JBJS.17.01245
2. Fassiotto, M., Simard, C., Sandborg, C., Valantine, H., & Raymond, J. (2018). An integrated career coaching and time-banking system promoting flexibility, wellness, and success: A pilot program at Stanford University School of Medicine. Academic Medicine, 93(6), 881–887. https://doi.org/10.1097/ACM.0000000000002081
3. Fortney, L., Luchterhand, C., Zakletskaia, L., Zgierska, A., & Rakel, D. (2013). Abbreviated mindfulness intervention for job satisfaction, quality of life, and compassion in primary care clinicians: A pilot study. Annals of Family Medicine, 11(5), 412–420. https://doi.org/10.1370/afm.1511
4. García, H., & Miralles, F. (2017). Ikigai: The Japanese secret to a long and happy life. Penguin Books.
5. Grischkan, J., George, B. P., Young, M. E., et al. (2022). Financial literacy and physician wellness: A systematic review. Journal of General Internal Medicine, 37(7), 1786–1793. https://doi.org/10.1007/s11606-021-07128-6
6. Hu, Y.-Y., Ellis, R. J., Hewitt, D. B., et al. (2019). Discrimination, abuse, harassment, and burnout in surgical residency training. New England Journal of Medicine, 381(18), 1741–1752. https://doi.org/10.1056/NEJMsa1903759
7. Koshy K., Limb C., Gundogan B., Whitehurst K., Jafree D.J. Reflective Practice in Health Care and How to Reflect Effectively. Int. J. Surg. Oncol. 2017;2:e20.

8. Panagioti, M., Panagopoulou, E., Bower, P., et al. (2017). Controlled interventions to reduce burnout in physicians: A systematic review and meta-analysis. JAMA Internal Medicine, 177(2), 195–205. https://doi.org/10.1001/jamainternmed.2016.7674

9. Rebar, A. L., Stanton, R., Geard, D., Short, C., Duncan, M. J., & Vandelanotte, C. (2015). A meta-analysis of the effect of physical exercise on depression and anxiety in non-clinical adult populations. Health Psychology Review, 9(2), 366–378. https://doi.org/10.1080/1743719 9.2014.915921

10. Scott, S. D., Hirschinger, L. E., Cox, K. R., et al. (2009). The natural history of recovery for the healthcare provider "second victim" after adverse patient events. Quality and Safety in Health Care, 18(5), 325–330. https://doi.org/10.1136/qshc.2009.032870

11. Shanafelt, T. D., Balch, C. M., Bechamps, G. J., et al. (2012). Burnout and career satisfaction among American surgeons. Annals of Surgery, 250(3), 463–471. https://doi.org/10.1097/ SLA.0b013e31817e0c8a

12. Szalados, J. E. (2007). Personal health and wellness of the practicing anesthesiologist: A review of the literature and strategies for success. Anesthesiology Clinics, 25(3), 627–646. https://doi.org/10.1016/j.anclin.2007.07.001

Chapter 39
Stronger with Every Cut: Lessons in Resilience

Amy Vertrees

Introduction

Any high-stakes career will require resilience. A recent Google search defined resilience as "the capacity to withstand or to recover quickly from difficulties" [1]. It is the ability to experience challenges, recover, adapt, and emerge stronger. Research on resilience focused first on how animals and then humans respond to painful stimuli. Experiments in the late 1960s discovered that when animals experienced pain and didn't have control over it, they just gave up. This was found to be true for humans, too, and in 1975, Donald Hiroto and Martin Seligman coined the term "learned helplessness" [2]. They later recognized that there is a normal distribution of reaction to painful stimuli. On one end, there is PTSD, depression, and suicide. The other end of the spectrum, people who also experienced a painful stimulus, seemed to be better off than they were before they started. Frederick Nietzsche coined the term "what doesn't kill you makes you stronger." Given the idea that everyone has the capability to choose their response, research focused on how to change the curve of response.

Resilience for women in surgery may look different from that of men, from other fields, and in her own career, as the stressors vary. Women in surgery have unique challenges, including gender biases, microaggressions, isolation, and work-life balance challenges. The challenges are not static; they change throughout her career, and strategies for resilience will need to change as well. The idea of resilience without understanding the meaning could lead to rejection of the idea. Suggesting resilience when you are beyond burned out may lead to a hostile response, if the assumption is that they are supposed to just deal with what happens or dismiss biases as acceptable. Resilience is not giving up, perpetuating a toxic culture, or not

A. Vertrees (✉)
Boss Business of Surgery Series, Columbia, TN, USA
e-mail: drvertrees@gmail.com

K. Yoon-Flannery et al. (eds.), *Women in Surgery*,
https://doi.org/10.1007/978-3-032-10971-2_39

213

fighting. Resilience is about creating a mindset that allows one to thrive in a high-stakes environment, identify and challenge biases, cultivate skills, advocate for change, and redefine success. Resilience is not something inherent; it is a skill that is developed over time after significant challenges.

Strategies for resilience must evolve with the career changes. Early career challenges in surgery are related to the draw of becoming a surgeon: it is hard, and not everyone can do it. The field of medicine, and especially surgery, is challenging due to the technical, cognitive, and emotional challenges. At first, it seems like the technical challenges would be the most significant, but over time, the ability to diagnose, choose the right operation (or not operate), and emotional challenges involving dealing with other strong personalities overshadow the technical challenges. What was initially incision, retraction, tissue handling, and efficient steps of the operation evolved into managing our insecurities, controlling other people's opinion about us, leading and inspiring others with similar insecurities, and the courage to move on after complications.

Many women may thrive early in their careers, as success is defined by a strong work ethic and gaining knowledge. Resilience involves developing endurance and survival strategies to deal with heavy workloads, challenging schedules, and exposure to gender biases. Resilience involves stamina, recovery, mentorship, and grit. Hard work is generally rewarded. That is great for the level at the time, with being perfect and people pleasing leading to success, but it creates the idea that problems can be solved by working hard and getting the answers right.

As women progress into clinical rotations with increased interactions with other people, biases are more evident [3]. In early surgery training, we are given "the hammer." Follow my orders, and the surgeon is in charge. Current society norms accept that from men in general, but society has a different unconscious expectation of women. What is modeled is certainty, firmness, and leading the team. Over time, this leads to validation in men and punishment in women [3]. Learning the same lessons, but the results are different, can be difficult to navigate for women, as the biases are not seen, and it seems more like a personal flaw. A difficult job becomes more challenging when the game changes. There is a subtle "you can't act in this way" that is internalized as "it's me, I'm the problem." Imposter syndrome can sneak in at this point, so even when the stimulus is gone, the doubt is generated internally and feeds itself.

When faced with challenges, it's common to fall back on strategies that have worked before. The idea that "if you just work hard enough, everything will be fine" starts to fall apart when you start interacting with other people. The learned responses of working hard as the solution could lead women to work much harder than their counterparts. The pressure to be perfect as the solution to the discomfort for the stressors and inconsistent treatment from bias leads to the perfectionist trap, and that discomfort could lead to maladaptive strategies like overworking and sacrificing the joys in life and turning to habits that relieve the pain but add to suffering, including alcohol, food, and "doomscrolling."

If perfectionist tendencies are not identified and managed, they can project onto other people and lead to doubt in them and within, fostering insecurity and leading to defensiveness. The inability to rebound from stress could spiral into "I am not capable or worthy of this… and neither are you" and jobs become a scary place where no one feels safe. Without intervention, burnout and exiting the profession could occur.

Martin Seligman, a psychologist who has studied resilience for decades, identified three ways people respond to setbacks known as the 3Ps of resilience: personalization, pervasiveness, and permanence [4]. When overwhelmed, there is a tendency to think that there is something wrong with us (personalization), that everyone feels that way about us (pervasiveness), and that it will never change (permanence). If the underlying causes of overworking and perfectionist thinking are not identified and managed, the result could be exiting the career or self-harm.

In mid-career, clinical competence and confidence come with experience, and the next challenges are often related to maintaining and defending competence and managing complications. Surgical decision-making often involves complexity, uncertainty, time management struggles, and challenging situations. Regret, shame, and feelings of inadequacy can be magnified after complications if not managed. Practical strategies include mindset shifts with coaching, therapy, mentorship, and a supportive network. Specific strategies include shame resilience as described by Brene Brown in "Daring Greatly." Reaching out to a trusted source is gaining strength from your community. Talking kindly to yourself is showing compassion. Owning the story allows you to own the ending and show your courage [5].

In addition to challenges at work, the balance of personal and professional goals, isolation, and the need for personal advocacy require specific skills to prevent overwhelm. Boundary setting is a necessary skill and involves a strategy of defining the boundary, communicating what the boundary is to those who need to know, and defining and executing a consequence if the boundary is violated. For example, work calls after hours will happen. Executing a successful boundary could be informing others that you do not accept calls after work hours, and you don't answer the calls when they call.

The end stages of a surgeon's career focus on legacy and transition. The mental shift required to be less hands-on to greater mentorship, teaching, and advising comes naturally to some and is met with resistance in others. It requires redefining professional identity and redefining success. The problem is that it doesn't feel simple, and the solution is breaking it down into steps that are simple. Professional coaching can help with targeted questions and simple, discrete steps to help in the transition. After a successful career with many challenges, turning pain into purpose could be the fourth P of resilience, as there is power in purpose, and the pain felt was not in vain. Resilience allows post-traumatic growth with wisdom, humility, and knowledge.

Resilience is resistance to stress, the ability to rebound, allowing growth and leaping forward. Women who can resist the internal and external stress are also likely to empower themselves. They learn more about who they are, because they are unwilling to be someone that they are not. The stress is about the stressor, and not about their ability and capability. Resilience involves managing burnout, emotional intelligence, conflict resolution, setting boundaries and priorities, resolving self-doubt, and focusing on self-care. By being more available to others, it's possible to share knowledge and experience. Seeing the exponential effect on the world is powerful and unlocks the secret to resilience: optimism. It's not me, it's not everywhere, it's not forever, and there is a reason for it.

Conclusion

Resilience is a necessary skill in a high-stakes environment. It is not merely enduring a challenge; it is becoming a better, more evolved, and authentic version of ourselves. As women surgeons progress through different career transitions, the challenges evolve from one of survival as an individual to strategic leadership in a system. Each level requires a different skill set and adaptation, which allows building personal growth, validation, meaningful connections, lasting change, and a legacy of exponential effect and lasting impact. Embracing challenges and the skills needed to adapt and recover in the dynamic evolution of her career will create the examples needed to empower the next generation of women in surgery.

References

1. https://www.google.com/search?q=resilience&rlz=1C5CHFA_enUS947US955&oq=resil&gs_lcrp=EgZjaHJvbWUqDggAEEUYJxg7GIAEGIoFMg4IABBFGCcYOxiABBiKBTIGCAEQRRg5MhAIAhAAGJECGLEDGIAEGIoFMg8IAxAAGEMYsQMYgAQYigUyDAgEEAAYQxiABBiKBTIGCAUQRRg9MgYIBhBFGDwyBggHEEUYPdIBCDQ1NDhqMGo3qAIAsAIA&sourceid=chrome&ie=UTF-8 Accessed 9 Feb 2025
2. Maier, S. F., & Seligman, M. E. (1976). Learned helplessness: Theory and evidence. *Journal of Experimental Psychology: General, 105*(1), 3–46. https://doi.org/10.1037/0096-3445.105.1.3 Accessed 9 Feb 2025
3. Bruce, A. N., Battista, A., Plankey, M. W., Johnson, L. B., & Marshall, M. B. (2015). Perceptions of gender-based discrimination during surgical training and practice. *OnlineMedical Education, 20*(1). https://doi.org/10.3402/meo.v20.25923
4. Seligman, M. E. P. (2025, Feb 9) Harvard business review. https://hbr.org/2011/04/building-resilience
5. Brown, B. (2015). *Daring Greatly.*

Chapter 40
When the System Fails: Maintaining Balance and Resilience

Amber Batool

Introduction

Surgery is not just a profession—it's an identity. And for many women, it is one we have fought hard to claim. We pour ourselves into the work, the training, the teaching, the leading. But what happens when the system around us starts to fall apart? When no amount of dedication can keep the wheels turning?

This chapter is not written from a place of having all the answers. It is written from the trenches—from the experience of watching a hospital decline, a residency program close, and a trauma system collapse, all while trying to keep going. I hope by sharing my story, other women in surgery will feel a little less alone. And maybe, just maybe, it will help us all learn to give ourselves a little more grace.

The Early Years: Hope and Hustle

I finished my fellowship in Surgical Critical Care at Cooper University Medical Center with the fire of purpose in my chest. I was ready to dive in—to care, to lead, to teach. My first job at Lancaster General Hospital felt like a dream start. But after only a year, family circumstances required me to leave. That was my first lesson in letting go of "the plan."

I soon joined Crozer Medical Center. It was a bustling, vibrant hospital with multiple specialties and an active trauma service. It had just been acquired by a for-profit company, and though we were cautiously optimistic, we didn't know how dramatically things would change.

A. Batool (✉)
Assistant Professor of Surgery, Drexel University College of Medicine, Philadelphia, PA, USA
e-mail: batool.amber@gmail.com

The Cracks Begin to Show

Then came COVID-19. The strain was unlike anything we had seen. Financial pressures tightened. PPE was scarce. And when many of our surgical partners hesitated to operate on COVID-positive patients, I—alongside my steadfast colleague Dr. Ratnasekera—kept operating. We didn't feel brave. We just knew our patients needed us.

Still, the cracks in the system were starting to show. As financial constraints intensified, institutional priorities began to shift. Certain service lines appeared to receive disproportionate support while others—equally vital to patient care—experienced gradual withdrawal of resources. It felt like a case of "robbing Peter to pay Paul." For trauma and surgical critical care, this meant navigating patient care with diminishing institutional backing.

At the same time, leadership transitions added another layer of complexity. With administrative turnover, relationships had to be rebuilt—often from scratch—and alignment on priorities was difficult to sustain. Advocating for trauma services in this environment required more than just clinical data or patient outcomes—it required diplomacy, persistence, and the ability to negotiate under pressure.

I developed these skills out of necessity. I began to reach out regularly to senior partners and trusted mentors, walking through difficult scenarios with them, seeking feedback, and learning how to present needs calmly and effectively. I learned that being composed and focused—even when advocating passionately—was often more effective than expressing frustration. Whether I was requesting additional trauma surgeon coverage, orthopedic support for trauma cases, or interventional radiology availability, I approached each conversation with preparation, transparency, and respect.

The Heartbreak of Residency Closure

Soon after I took over, things got worse. Two sister hospitals in our network closed, surgical volumes plummeted, and our faculty numbers shrank. Our residents—understandably upset—expressed their frustration. The ACGME survey results were scathing. Some of the criticism felt fair, but some of it felt personal, even retaliatory.

We underwent a brutal ACGME site visit. I worked day and night to prepare. I carried it all—every criticism, every complaint—as if it were my fault. We appealed the ACGME decision and met with lawyers regularly. We compiled a detailed, evidence-based response to every allegation. But despite our efforts, the decision remained unchanged.

That moment broke something in me. I had tried so hard. I took it all so personally. But with time, I learned something invaluable: you can give your whole heart and still lose. And that doesn't make you a failure. It just means you are human.

In those dark moments, I reached out to mentors—women and men I trusted for their wisdom and grace. Their support reminded me to zoom out. They helped me separate my worth from the outcome. I also leaned on my partners and friends, who served as sounding boards, cheerleaders, and truth-tellers. Those conversations were not just therapeutic—they were strategic.

I realized I couldn't lead by simply reacting. I had to pivot from frustration to solutions. Instead of focusing solely on the problems, I asked myself: What can we try? Who can help? What can we fix today? I learned to be diplomatic, to present ideas in a way that brought others along, and to listen carefully when others offered feedback—even when it was hard to hear.

I brought the entire group together—faculty, staff, and residents—and was honest with them. I didn't pretend to have all the answers. I asked for their input. I made them part of the process. That collective approach didn't fix everything, but it changed the tone. It turned helplessness into shared ownership.

There was still a silver lining. All of my residents transitioned into other programs. My chief residents graduated on time, passed their boards, and went on to flourish. That was a win I still carry with pride. For me, that was success.

A New Role, A New Set of Challenges

After the residency closed, I was offered the role of Trauma Medical Director. I accepted, knowing the road ahead would be steep. We had a Pennsylvania Trauma Systems Foundation (PTSF) survey in less than a year—preparation should have started months earlier. We were down to three full-time trauma surgeons, soon to be two. Most of our support came from locums and per diems. Our mid-level coverage was shrinking fast.

I knew we didn't have what we needed. But I also knew I had to try.

So, we pushed ahead. I again reached out to colleagues around the country for advice. I asked mentors how they had approached surveys with limited support. Their guidance helped me stay grounded and creative. We made changes, we worked with what we had.

I had to fight to get our vendors paid on time so we could maintain vital trauma services—including locums trauma surgeons, orthopedic trauma support, and interventional radiology. These services were essential to maintaining our trauma designation, and I had to advocate fiercely for every one of them.

At the same time, I worked on the culture. Implementing change—especially culture change—is hard. In a fractured system, it is even harder. I built relationships across departments, established trust, and motivated a weary team. I invited feedback and made people feel heard. I reminded myself daily: *My circumstances are not a reflection of my effort.* That mantra became my lifeline.

Then Came the Bankruptcy

Just when it seemed things could not get worse, our parent company filed for bankruptcy.

Despite the looming uncertainty, we never paused our efforts. We were a critical access point in a socioeconomically disadvantaged community, and we knew our patients would continue to come—regardless of corporate restructuring. They depended on us, and we were committed to showing up.

Even with limited resources, we continued preparing for the trauma survey. We maintained open communication with the PTSF, informing them of our institutional challenges and seeking their input on how to remain compliant with trauma standards. Their collaboration allowed us to stay focused on what mattered most: delivering the highest quality of care under the circumstances we faced.

Securing key resources—such as locum trauma surgeons, orthopedic trauma support, and interventional radiology—required constant advocacy. At times, I found myself not just requesting but pleading for what was necessary to uphold care standards. But I did so with a steady voice, rooted in data, compassion, and a clear understanding of the stakes.

Those last few weeks were unbearable. Every shift felt like a goodbye. Telling my team they were terminated because our trauma system no longer existed was one of the hardest things I've ever had to do.

Yet, through it all, I continued to advocate for patient care, support my staff, and provide mentorship. I brought the team together again—not to give them false hope, but to help us close with dignity. I let them speak, cry, question. We processed it together. That transparency, I believe, softened the blow.

This chapter of my life taught me that leadership in medicine is not just about guiding others through success—but about standing steady in the storm.

Looking back, I had opportunities to leave the system. But I made the decision to stay. And I don't regret it. I was where I needed to be. That experience shaped me. It made me stronger. It made me more grounded. And it deepened my appreciation for what we often take for granted—resources, infrastructure, stability, and each other.

As the hospital closed, I found something I had not expected: clarity. I had endured so much, but I was still standing. And in that, I found resilience.

When a system fails, it is easy to feel like you have failed too. But you haven't. Not if you kept trying. Not if you showed up. Not if you led with integrity, even when no one was watching.

This chapter is for every woman who has stayed in a broken system just long enough to make sure it didn't collapse on someone else.

You are not alone. And your resilience is not invisible.

Chapter 41
Being a Male Mentor to a Female Surgeon

Marc A. Neff

I am honored and blessed to be an accomplished male mentor to so many remarkable and dynamic women in my career. I have been a teaching attending since 2003, when I started my surgical career at Crozer-Chester Medical Center after fellowship. At a low estimate, I've been a mentor to over 50 female residents, at a high, over 100. And that doesn't include the female medical students, physician assistant students, and rotating interns I've been fortunate enough to interact with. I thought of many ways to start this chapter, even using the AI "Copilot" to come up with some appropriate topics to cover. The list was daunting, everything from understanding gender dynamics in surgical training to addressing implicit bias and promoting inclusivity.

For most of my career, in teaching women, I have tried to recognize the challenges faced by women in surgery. Be sensitive to them. I believe the male mentors play a significant role in supporting the development of female surgeons. For this chapter, I will focus on building trust and respect in the mentor-mentee relationship, the role of male mentors in supporting female surgeons, and creating a supportive and inclusive surgical environment.

Building trust and respect in the mentor-mentee relationship when the mentor is male and the mentee is female requires careful attention to open communication, role modeling, and confidentiality. Regarding open communication in the mentor/mentee relationship, both participants should feel comfortable discussing concerns and expectations. I can remember one specific mentee where we sat down, and both took notes on each other's perspectives, and this became the basis of our regular check-ins. Furthermore, male mentors need to strive to be positive role models demonstrating integrity and professionalism. Proper behavior is leading by example. Lastly, I have found that maintaining confidentiality is vital to allow the mentee to

M. A. Neff (✉)
Center for Surgical Weight Loss, Jefferson Health New Jersey, Cherry Hill, NJ, USA
e-mail: mneffyhs@aol.com

K. Yoon-Flannery et al. (eds.), *Women in Surgery*,
https://doi.org/10.1007/978-3-032-10971-2_41

221

feel secure in sharing thoughts and concerns. One mentee I can recall sat with me and vented about their crumbling relationship with their husband. The confidential support and encouragement I offered, I like to think, empowered the female mentee to survive and thrive through this traumatic episode in their life.

The role of male mentors in supporting female surgeons includes guidance and expertise, advocacy and sponsorship, and networking opportunities. Whether male or female, the role of the mentor is always to provide insight in navigating the complexity of the medical field through sharing their knowledge and experience. And, as we all know, wisdom comes from experience, the best wisdom, from the worst experience. Furthermore, surgery is still a male-dominated field, and the male mentor can sponsor female surgeons for opportunities in research, presentations, and even leadership roles. I've been uniquely blessed to connect several young female surgeons with my contacts at Springer for their own book developments. Finally, male mentors may have established professional networks that could provide invaluable support for the young female surgeon in defining their career trajectory. As a member of the Philadelphia Academy of Surgery, I was able to help two remarkably talented female surgeons access this prestigious organization, and I am proud to say, both are on their way to becoming officers.

Creating a supportive and inclusive surgical environment is critical to maximizing the potential of our future female surgeons. Keys to this goal are *ensuring equal opportunities, addressing work-life balance, and recognizing and celebrating achievements*. With regards to ensuring equal opportunities, male mentors must ensure equal access to all residents in training, regardless of sex or gender, for education. This includes distribution of surgical cases; in fact, many times, I have found the female surgical resident to approach the surgical case they scrub on with me with a more balanced and less cowboy approach to the task at hand. Work-life balance must be addressed, as still, even today, many women need support when pregnant or breastfeeding, and flexible work arrangements and resources for childcare/parental leave policies should be considered. I vividly recall contaminating my 9-month pregnant resident, who refused to sit down at the end of the case because she felt it was important to close the incisions herself. Finally, it may be suggested that it is favoritism, but the importance of the celebration of achievements in public cannot be understated. Acknowledgment of awards, presentations, and promotions in public creates a culture of positivity, focused on positive reinforcement, appreciation, and respect.

The future of male mentors and women in surgery lies in continued efforts to promote diversity, inclusivity, and support. By fostering strong mentorship relationships, we can create a more equitable and diverse, and I would argue, a more balanced and successful surgical community.

Chapter 42
When Your Patient Dies

Kahyun Yoon-Flannery

"Just let me know when it's my time—I don't want to hear it from someone else other than you."

Lisa asked me for this favor as we were talking about how her cancer was progressing. I had only diagnosed her with inflammatory breast cancer fewer than 2 years ago. We went through a vigorous round of chemotherapy at first. I say we, not she, because she involved me in every aspect of her care, more than any other patient ever had asked of me. She asked me for "just the right chemo doctor you can think of" and let me know of every bout of nausea or fatigue throughout her treatment, all the while telling all of us, "we are going to beat this". When we got her pathology back from her surgery, and I had to tell her that the chemotherapy had not worked as well as we had hoped, she did not lose hope. In fact, she gained it for all of us. "I know you always do your best, so I know I'm going to be fine"—these were her words as I shook away any doubt I had in all of our data on how patients fare based on the presence of residual cancer after neoadjuvant chemotherapy.

When she called me over a weekend, telling me she was yellow—I knew the day I was dreading was here faster than all of us had predicted. She told me that she looked like a crazy doll—yellow and swollen in her belly. Even before I sent her to the emergency room, I knew. I knew that the cancer had progressed, far from her breast that I had already removed, to her liver, riddling it all throughout, hindering its own natural ways to heal. She didn't blame me, God, or anyone. She told me to tell her what to do, and that she would do it. Whatever I told her, she was going to do it because she had to be here for her husband. So I gritted my teeth once again, conferred with her medical oncologist, and we formulated a plan for her second line of therapy.

K. Yoon-Flannery (✉)
Chief of Women's Cancer Services, Chief of Breast Surgery, Atlanticare Regional Medical Center, Egg Harbor Township, NJ, USA
e-mail: kay.yoonflannery@gmail.com

K. Yoon-Flannery et al. (eds.), *Women in Surgery*,
https://doi.org/10.1007/978-3-032-10971-2_42

After her return home, she was okay for a few weeks. Waiting for the "pre-authorization" to take place for her next line of treatment. And all the more texting me to check in, more with me and not for me to check in with her. "If you think we got this, I know we did." She fainted at home, which prompted another ride in the ambulance. She woke up, just as her brain MRI result came back, ever so efficiently through the patient portal, and she texted me as I was crossing the street to enter the ER to see her. "Is this shit in my brain too?" I had not even had a chance to look at her MRI—and I had to tell her in that room in the crazy busy ER that not only did the cancer spread into her abdomen but into her brain as well. I think I wanted her to blame me just a little bit, or at least tell me. She never wavered in her belief in her surgeon. The surgeon who had become her friend and confidante over this cancer and life in general, she would never bring herself to doubt her abilities.

In the next week, I saw an ugly progression. Although I had seen a few, thankfully, of my patients progress to having metastatic breast cancer, usually this would happen over the years. Sometimes cancer progresses too slowly, if you could even imagine that, and allows too much idle time for patients to suffer. Lisa's cancer wasn't like one of those. Just a few days after she texted me about her MRI results, I texted her before I could go back to the hospital to see how she was doing. No response. I knew in my heart something was wrong. She would answer me day or night, or maybe it was me answering her day or night, it's hard to see—but she would always respond to my question. When my text went unanswered, I knew the time was already here too fast.

I went into her room. She must have been tossing and turning in that patient room all night. The bedding was a "hot mess," as she would tell me. She was as yellow as a traffic light—as she once told me. "Lisa?" I asked. "Do you know who I am?" I asked, afraid of what she might say in her delirium that came way too fast. Then she answered me, "Of course, I know who you are. You are Dr. Flannery, my best friend who saved my life. I will never forget you."

As a breast surgeon, fortunately for us, we don't get a lot of opportunities to deal with end-of-life discussions and decisions. First of all, as I like to boast to my residents and students, most breast cancer patients that surgeons see are at an early stage, thankfully. And in those unfortunate circumstances where our patients do progress, usually the discussion happens with a medical oncologist, and we are spared the heartache. For Lisa, that discussion couldn't be had by anyone else but me. I called her husband after I stepped out of her room, and told him it was time for us to bring her home.

It has been so many years since that Sunday I received her husband's text saying she was gone. Reflecting on Lisa's journey, I am reminded of the humbling power of cancer—its capacity to grow and spread in devastating bursts that defy our best medical efforts. Our patients place immense faith in us, often more than we sometimes feel we deserve. This trust is not merely medical but deeply personal, binding patients and doctors in a shared human experience that transcends medicine.

Lisa's trust in me and her unwavering faith despite her progressing cancer have been a profound influence on my practice. It drives home the importance of my work, not just in the technical execution of surgical procedures but in the compassionate care I must provide. Each patient's trust allows me to continue, pushing me forward even when it seems impossible.

Chapter 43
A Nurse Practitioner's Perspective Over 20 Years

Hannah M. Sadek

About Me/Who Am I?

When I was asked to write a chapter for a book about women in surgery, I was extremely flattered to be included in such an endeavor. I was asked to reflect on the last 20 years of my experience in medicine and describe my perspective on how medicine has changed for women in surgery. Of course, such a request had me reflect on my own career as well as those individuals along the way that I have known and grown with. I have worked in healthcare for over 20 years, as both a nurse and a nurse practitioner, working in the inpatient and outpatient settings in cardiac surgery, trauma surgery, emergency general surgery, and the surgical intensive care unit. I have seen healthcare from multiple perspectives over a long period of time and have been witness to many practices and cultural changes. As a nurse, I have taught both formally in nursing school and as a preceptor and mentor in the hospital setting. I am known for high standards in patient care, communication, and collaboration. I have been a nurse practitioner for 11 years, and my responsibilities, in addition to direct patient care and stabilization, include mentoring, hiring, and onboarding advanced practice providers (APPs). One of my main goals is onboarding and cross-training to ensure that all APPs in my group are proficient in stabilizing and advancing patients along the continuum of care from the trauma bay to the ICU to the wards and eventual discharge. The training is thorough and details all phases from trauma stabilization to appropriate critical resuscitation to safe discharge. In addition, I play an integral role in supporting and training general surgery, emergency medicine, anesthesia residents, and medical students during their ICU rotations.

H. M. Sadek (✉)
Division of Acute Care Surgical Services, Virginia Commonwealth University Health, Richmond, VA, USA
e-mail: hannahsadek@gmail.com

© The Author(s), under exclusive license to Springer Nature Switzerland AG 2026
K. Yoon-Flannery et al. (eds.), *Women in Surgery*,
https://doi.org/10.1007/978-3-032-10971-2_43

In my time as a nurse and as a nurse practitioner, I have watched the progression and have prided myself on being a role model, a source of support, and a mentor to many generations of nurses, medical students, surgical residents, critical care fellows, and attending physicians.

Change in Culture

From my own perspective as a female APP in the surgical field, I have seen vast changes in my role alone. When I was first training to be a nurse practitioner, the majority of NPs were female, and our role was to "help" in the ICU. The surgical residents assumed care of the majority of the patients, and the nurse practitioners helped on rounds, took a few patients, and slightly eased the burden. Currently, due to ACGME requirements and the evolution of advanced practice providers, nurse practitioners and physician assistants (APPs) have a primary role in the management of the intensive care unit, and some units in the country are strictly run by APPs. Nurses feel more comfortable today speaking up to participate in the plan and in the decision-making aspect of patient care. Both nursing and advanced practice provider practices were once female-dominated, and now there are many males in these roles.

Beyond reflecting on my own experience, I used writing this chapter as an opportunity to touch base with and interview nurses, APPs, students, surgical residents, and surgeons I worked with over the decades. I then categorized them into those who have worked for more than 20 years, 10 to 20 years, 5 to 10 years, and less than 5 years. Reminiscing with friends who have been surgeons for more than 20 years, they recall that it was a male-dominated field and very difficult to succeed as a female surgeon. Surprisingly, they report their biggest obstacles today are resistance from novice and younger female hospital staff and an aggression/hazing that seems to go along with being a female surgeon. In contrast, when discussing differences in training and treatment with surgeons less than 5 years of experience and female surgical residents, they feel that their programs were heavily female-dominated, and they have not only been extremely supported by their male leaders, but most have male surgeon mentors. In fact, several of the younger surgeons I spoke with say that when they struggled for different reasons and thought of quitting their training program, it was their male leaders who talked them out of it and went above and beyond to help them succeed.

The differences over time are striking to me, with the more experienced female surgeons feeling that they had to fight for their place and the novice female surgeons feeling that they have not had limited opportunities due to their gender. While this change in culture was wonderful to hear, I also was disappointed to learn of many ongoing struggles. Interestingly, across the timeline and the country, female surgeons and APPs still feel that they need to get "buy-in" from their nursing and ancillary staff and have to continue to work harder to earn the credibility that their male counterparts win more easily. In fact, in speaking with both surgeons and APPs, universally, many have inadvertently found out that their male counterparts have higher salaries. According to the Association of Women Surgeons, female surgeons earn 8% less than their male counterparts, and the pay disparity widens over time, affecting both immediate compensation and retirement. Also, a quick literature review showed similar trends for RNs, NPs, and PAs [3, 4].

Another common grievance that I found in my conversations is that there is a feeling that their requests are not taken seriously, and there is reprimand when advocating for either position or compensation. A surgeon who has been in her practice for over 5 years shared with me that her requested operating room days were given to a new male part-time surgeon to accommodate his schedule, and more concerning, that she was told there were no salary negotiations for the upcoming contract, but that the same part-time surgeon was waiting for his updated contract with his negotiated raise. Speaking to both APPs and MDs yielded many similarly disappointing stories.

What Is Needed

While I was very happy to hear the experience changes for younger female surgeons, it seems that more work is needed on multiple fronts. There is a consensus that there is ongoing gender bias, that leadership positions continue to be predominantly male occupied, that there is an ongoing pay gap, and that there needs to be more investment in work/life balance.

The gender bias is deeply ingrained and will likely take generations to change. However, this does not preclude the responsibility for ongoing efforts in this area. As we evolve and we become more mindful of diversity, equity, and inclusion, we should include more rigorous gender bias training along with our DEI initiatives. A unified message from female surgeons and practitioners is that they continuously have to adjust their style and provide extensive explanations to get cooperation for their plans. I received interesting feedback about women in leadership, and the style has to be one of collaboration and asking for permission to succeed. The consensus from everyone I spoke with is that women have to act more deferentially towards nurses, learners, and ancillary staff than men to achieve the same outcomes. In addition, the women leaders felt that they had to tailor their methods in that, before meaningful feedback, they had to give positive affirmation, so it would be received well. Sadly, even the younger women interviewed do feel that they have to "be better" to make it.

Impressive initiatives such as the Athena Scientific Women's Academic Network (SWAN) Charter in 2005 were set up for just this reason to transform gender equality [2]. It is a crucial responsibility to change expectations in this regard, and the conversations regarding gender bias have to remain at the forefront and transparent to affect bias literacy. Leadership positions continue to be male-dominated. While a few have been self-promoted, the majority of the female surgical leaders I have spoken with have had true sponsorship by male senior surgeons. Whether it is through mentorship, sponsorship, or formally increasing professional development opportunities for women, more focus needs to be invested to create pathways for female surgeon leadership [1].

From RNs to APPs to MDs, there is a known pay gap between male and female practitioners. Administrative departments need to be held accountable and have transparent reporting in terms of gender differences in salary structure. The topic of gender-based pay difference requires a zero-tolerance policy if there is to be a resolution of this issue [3, 4].

In terms of family planning, scheduling accommodations for both males and females would make this more feasible. I assisted one female surgeon in advocating to no longer work 24-hour shifts in her last trimester of pregnancy. There is extensive data that female surgeons have issues with fertility, healthy pregnancy, and birth complications due to stress and work hours. In addition, as we move towards a more wellness model in medicine, there could be more collaboration for work schedules that accommodate family planning and appropriate family time [1].

I believe that changing the focus is possible from many perspectives. On a personal note, as I have worked in medicine for multiple generations of learners, I have had to change my own approach to stay connected and effective. One approach that helped me extensively more than a decade ago was exploring the business model of mission and externally focused versus self-focused goals. The mission-based mindset shifts the goals to a shared purpose and a collective goal, prioritizing focus on a collaborative effort. Staying in this mindset helps shift from the ego and has us invested in the success of the whole group, and I have found improves outcomes from team dynamics to patient care. Training to include this concept can help bridge many differences, including gender bias. Although changes have been made over the decades, more expectations and transparency, and training on multiple fronts are needed to work towards gender equality, healthy workplaces, and equitable treatment.

References

1. Ferrari, L., Mari, V., Parini, S., Capelli, G., Tacconi, G., Chessa, A., … Spolverato, G. (2022). Discrimination toward women in surgery: a systematic scoping review. *Annals of Surgery*, *276*(1), 1–8.
2. Ovseiko, P. V., Chapple, A., Edmunds, L. D., & Ziebland, S. (2017). Advancing gender equality through the Athena SWAN Charter for Women in Science: an exploratory study of women's and men's perceptions. *Health research policy and systems*, *15*, 1–13.
3. Lin, J. C., Bowser, K. E., Drudi, L. M., DiLosa, K. L., & Yi, J. (2021). Equal pay for equal work: disparities in compensation in vascular surgery. *Journal of vascular surgery*, *74*(2), 21S–28S.
4. Greene, J., El-Banna, M. M., Briggs, L. A., & Park, J. (2017). Gender differences in nurse practitioner salaries. *Journal of the American Association of Nurse Practitioners*, *29*(11), 667–672.
5. Gauci, P., Elmir, R., O'reilly, K., & Peters, K. (2022). Women's experiences of workplace gender discrimination in nursing: An integrative review. *Collegian*, *29*(2), 188–200.

Chapter 44
Whistleblowing Within Your Health System

"Primum non nocere"

Beth B. DuPree

Introduction

As physicians, we take an oath to first do no harm as we practice the art and science of medicine. I took that oath quite seriously as I am certain that the majority of physicians do as well. Never could I have predicted that during my surgical career, I would be in a position where a private physician group, health system administrators, and hospital board trustees would choose to ignore a significant patient safety issue, choosing opacity over transparency. If you find yourself in a similar position, you likely will doubt yourself and what you are seeing. When you recognize that you are the sane one, aka the adult in the room, you need to act. I have served as the Chair of Quality and Reliability for Redeemer Health System for years, so I was acutely aware of how to raise a quality concern. As surgeons, we are trained to take responsibility for every aspect of our patients' care, and being certain in what we see right in front of us is paramount to providing the best care. When you are placed in a situation where you follow all the rules to correct a ship that has gone off course, you may be placed in a position where your only recourse is to become a *"whistleblower."*

Once You See, You Cannot Unsee!

In the fall of 2017, I started a position as an employed breast cancer surgeon tasked with assembling a team to create a state-of-the-art breast cancer center for a large independent health system. I did a gap analysis in the year before I became

B. B. DuPree (✉)
Redeemer Health, Southampton, PA, USA
e-mail: bbdmouth@gmail.com

K. Yoon-Flannery et al. (eds.), *Women in Surgery*,
https://doi.org/10.1007/978-3-032-10971-2_44

employed, and so I was aware that there were countless opportunities for improvement, but that is why they were hiring an experienced breast cancer surgeon. If they had had all the pieces and parts in place, hiring a leader to head up an NAPBC (National Accreditation Program for Breast Centers) breast health program would not have been needed. Hindsight is 20/20, and in retrospect, I should have anticipated that I could possibly be entering a hostile work environment. The private radiology group, the solitary provider for the entire health system, would not engage with me prior to my arrival. I had requested practice data to created a comprehensive gap analysis, as I was trying to determine the needs for the three-campus hospital system. Within the first 4 weeks in practice, my rose-colored glasses developed crystal clarity when a quality concern fell on deaf ears and was completely discounted at many levels through many levels of the health system.

The first patient of concern, that I evaluated in the office, was sent to me by her primary care physician for an abnormal lymph node on her MRI on the left side, where she had previously had a mastectomy for cancer over a decade earlier. Pat had been receiving annual mammograms, including 3D tomosynthesis films, for the prior 2–3 years of her right breast. She had an abnormal lymph node on her left side where her prior cancer had been treated with a left mastectomy. Before I went to examine the patient I reviewed several years of her films, as I always do with a new patient. I could not believe what I saw with my own eyes on her imaging. She had imaging evidence of a locally advanced right breast cancer, larger than a lemon, that had been clearly visible and evolving for the past 5–6 years, including thickening of the skin and retraction of the breast. I reread the MRI and mammogram reports, thinking that the dictations must have been somehow confused with another patient, but NO, several radiologists missed the obvious cancer as it progressed, even dictating erroneously that she had radiation changes in the skin of her right breast. (The right breast that never had cancer treatment!) Mind-blowing to say the least!!

My quality nightmare had officially begun. I reached out to the radiologists directly to discuss my concerns about several cases, including Pat's, and repeatedly refused a meeting. I went to the administration, and they suggested submitting RDEs (Remote Data Entry, the official quality system), and since I was beyond busy with the practice, the Oncology administrator submitted the first eight cases where I had concerns for review. The quality process took several months, and the committee came back that there were NO concerns based upon the "radiology groups" internal review. I went to the COO of the hospital and requested an external review with dedicated breast imagers, but got a "general radiology review granted." My request was rewarded by being bullied and berated by the radiology group over Zoom for having doubted their interpretations. The COO and chair of the quality committee heard the concern in my voice during that meeting and after my insistence sent several cases for external review. The external review came back with significant concerns, and by this time, I had upwards of 40 cases that were concerning to me for a delay in diagnosis. The 3D tomosynthesis (tomo) had been installed in the health system since 2016, and these cancers were easily visible on the "tomo" images. I then requested an external review with "dedicated breast imagers." This process took nearly 18 months from my arrival at the health system. The radiology group had added a dedicated breast imager, and her story of why she chose to join that group without really knowing their quality is the subject of a future Netflix documentary.

The external breast imager specific review was returned to the health system, and what was shared with me by the CMO was that they felt it was the most egregious review they had ever completed. This prompted an internal review of over 6000 images read as negative previously. Our 3 dedicated imagers in the fall of 2019 identified 27 additional cancers that had been overlooked by the general radiologists readings as well as several atypical lesions that required excision. The hospital COO who ordered the review was let go on a Friday in relatively close proximity to the time the review was released, but it was "unrelated". One of the radiologists responsible for a large number of missed cancers was allowed to resign and was not reported to the medical board by the hospital despite the quality issues. We, the breast imagers and breast care team, who were responsible for the health system attaining NAPBC accredited in December 2019, were assured that the health system was going to disclose the issue we identified, hold the radiology group accountable, and allow us to move forward with a high-quality program. Then COVID-19 made its appearance and the leadership's decision to not to disclose and not hold anyone accountable lead to a perpetual hostile environment for the dedicated breast imagers, my staff, and me.

I made the decision to resign from the health system in January 2020, after beginning my healing process for the PTSD that I believe they were responsible for perpetuating. The COVID-19 pandemic hit, and the world came to a standstill. Simultaneously, my breast surgeon colleague, who was starting in the area and could have assumed the care of my patients, nearly died and became a permanently disabled from a car accident in May 2020. I actually ended up becoming responsible for all of her patients. My commitment to her patients and my patients superseded my need to leave a toxic health system and work environment. It was simply a matter of time until I could extricate myself from the toxicity.

My colleagues and I, after no action from the health system leadership and health system board, reported our concerns to the medical board, the state Attorney General's office, and eventually the federal Attorney General's office. In the fall of 2022, the story appeared in the local newspaper and then nationally on the NBC Nightly News in October 2022. After nearly 5 years of investigation, surveillance, and data evaluation, we elected to drop the case as attaining the electronic data, aka. keystroke tracking of image reviews to prove any wrong doing, appeared nearly impossible. The bureaucracy was too much. Despite our trying to demand accountability for what had transpired, we have had to move on. I have healed this traumatic chapter years ago and could have stayed in the health system being paid very well, but I would have lost my integrity, and that's really all we have at the end of each day.

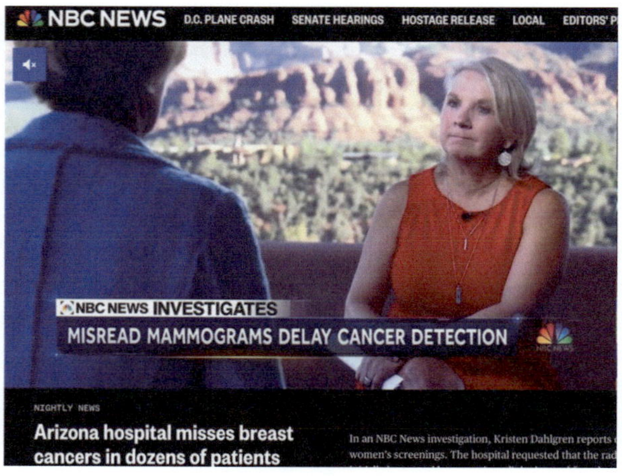

https://www.nbcnews.com/nightly-news/video/arizona-hospital-misses-breast-cancers-in-dozens-of-patients-151541829786

The financial and professional costs of whistleblowing can be huge and extend far beyond your personal sacrifices. They can include the loss of your income and your career, as well as the loss of the ability to follow up with your patients, leaving you feeling as though you have abandoned them post-surgery. PTSD as a result of working in a hostile work environment and feeling complicit in hiding the truth from patients is real. When your employer tells you that you cannot reveal a delay in diagnosis to a patient even if they ask "was this seen on my prior mammogram?" you experience a moral injury. When you are told to call risk management and have them talk to the patient you will feel handcuffed by administration. There was an entire army of doctors and healthcare professionals pushing for quality care who knew what had been going on in breast imaging, and what we wanted was account-ability and transparence and they wanted from all of us was silence.

At the end of the day, you need to be able to sleep at night and live with yourself, not simply professionally but personally. When you are essentially telling your health system that their "baby is ugly" and they turn a blind eye, your only recourse is to hold that baby up in public via the news, in front of the Attorney General's Office and State Medical Society and say, "SEE WHAT HAPPENED HERE." I was powerless to determine the results of blowing the whistle, but I now sleep well at night knowing that had I not moved to Arizona, when I did, many women could still have cancer in their breasts, not identified on breast imaging.

It is a shame how all of this unfolded, as all we asked for was honesty and trans-parency for our affected patients and the community. We felt that we deserved an in-depth investigation into additional images from the private practice radiologists and follow through, providing quality care.

The collateral damage was the resignation of two talented breast surgeons, four dedicated breast imagers, two medical oncologists, several nurse practitioners, nurse navigators, mammography technicians and ultrasound technicians, oncology administrators, and the journalist who broke the story locally in Sedona. I resigned my position in December 2021, as the health system was unwilling to be accountable and hold others accountable. I believe that they chose to just sweep these issues under the rug using the COVID-19 pandemic as cover believing no one would take notice. Other people's behavior is beyond your control, but choosing to accept their behavior will reflect badly on you.

Index

© The Editor(s) (if applicable) and The Author(s), under exclusive license to
Springer Nature Switzerland AG 2026
K. Yoon-Flannery et al. (eds.), *Women in Surgery*,
https://doi.org/10.1007/978-3-032-10971-2